J. Orley, W. Kuyken (Eds.)

Quality of Life Assessment: International Perspectives

Proceedings of the Joint-Meeting Organized by the World Health Organization and the Fondation IPSEN in Paris, July 2 - 3, 1993

With 4 Figures and 25 Tables

Springer-Verlag
Berlin Heidelberg New York
London Paris Tokyo
Hong Kong Barcelona Budapest

John Orley, M. D.
Willem Kuyken, Ph. D.

Division of Mental Health
World Health Organization
CH-1211 Geneva 27 / Switzerland

ISBN-13: 978-3-642-79125-3 e-ISBN-13: 978-3-642-79123-9
DOI:10.1007/ 978-3-642-79123-9

Library of Congress Cataloging-in-Publication Data. Quality of life assessment: international perspectives: proceedings of the joint-meeting organized by the World Health Organization and the Foundation IPSEN in paris, July 2–3, 1993 / J. Orley, W. Kuyken (eds.).
Includes bibliographical references and index.

1. Quality of life – Evaluation – Congresses. 2. Health status indicators – Congresses. I. Orley, J. (John), 1937– . II. Kuyken, W. (Willem), 1968– . III. World Health Organization. IV. Foundation IPSEN pour la recherche thérapeutique.

Softcover reprint of the hardcover 1st edition 1994

Typesetting: K+V Fotosatz, Beerfelden
SPIN: 10077627 27/3020-5 4 3 2 1 0 – Printed on acid-free paper

Preface

Considerable data and expertise have accumulated in the assessment of quality of life, but to date this assessment has largely been restricted to the development of instruments that are used only in the setting in which they were developed. The chapters of this book, taken together, apply this expertise to a relatively new area: international quality of life assessment, that is to say, considering quality of life from an international perspective, and developing methods for the assessment of quality of life that can be used in more than one cultural setting.

The World Health Organization (WHO) initiatives in the area of international quality of life assessment arose for several compelling reasons. The World Health Organization has a commitment to equitable and accessible health care for all. This commitment refers not only to health in its narrow sense of the absence of disease and impairment, but to health as a state of physical, mental and social well-being. Disease and impairment affect not just the physical domain of life but also a person's psychological state, level of independence and social relationships. This is a reality not yet fully reflected in health care settings. The broadening in focus in the measurement of health to include indicators which address this more holistic sense of health is a welcome emerging trend.

The primary aim of any health intervention is to maximise health and minimise disease, thereby enhancing patients' quality of life. At regional, national and international levels, quality of life data can be used in planning health policy, evaluating policy changes and auditing existing health services so that the concerns of patients are central to the process.

Furthermore, international quality of life data will enable research that can yield a more complete picture of the nature of disease. As an awareness of the ways in which disease and impairment impact on patients' quality of life grows among health personnel, the interaction between patients and health personnel will evolve to give more meaning and fulfilment to the health practitioner, and should lead to the patient being provided with more comprehensive care. Because an assessment is carried out which addresses patient's concerns in a broad range of areas, patients themselves may find the health care they receive more meaningful.

In spite of these many applications of quality of life data at international, as well as national, levels, there are as yet no standardised and validated ways of assessing quality of life across cultural and national boundaries.

The Assessment Challenge

In recent decades numerous assessments of the effects of disease and impairment have been developed, e.g., disability measures, functional status scales, activities of daily living checklists, psychological distress scales and perceived health scales. Some excellent measures for the assessment of the impact of disease and impairment on quality of life have also been developed in recent years, and extensively validated. However, to date these have been developed and used for the most part in single cultural settings. The assessment challenge, then, lies in applying the extensive data and expertise that have accumulated in the development of national quality of life measures to an international perspective on quality of life, and the development of an international quality of life assessment.

Sartorius and Kuyken outline some of the issues involved in translating health status measures for use in another culture/language region, and present a translation method that has been extensively used in international studies coordinated by WHO. Patrick and his colleagues describe the further step in developing international quality of life measures, the field testing of a new language version to assess its reliability, validity and responsiveness in different language versions. Bullinger describes a number of criteria that should be addressed in establishing whether different language/culture versions of an instrument are in fact equivalent. She goes on to discuss these criteria and to demonstrate their usefulness in relation to work on the translation into several languages of the USA Medical Outcomes Study Short Form 36 item measure of perceived health/disability. The WHOQOL Group close this section of the book with a description of the methodology and progress to date in the WHO project to develop an international quality of life assessment instrument (the WHOQOL), that will be both sensitive to the settings in which it is developed but also yield scores that are comparable between cultures.

These four chapters taken together begin to address the challenge of cross-cultural quality of life assessment. To obtain answers to questions about quality of life that are meaningful and comparable across cultures requires innovative methods and techniques. The considered development of these methods will take some time, but the data they will yield are likely to be fascinating, valuable and innovative.

Perspectives on Quality of Life

Quality of life is a term understood differently by workers in the many professions for whom it is relevant. Fox-Rushby demonstrates the important and far reaching implications of quality of life data in addressing the health economics questions, "Are limited resources used in the best possible ways?" The indices of health used to answer this question have increasingly begun to include quality of life measures, and the algorithms for combining and using these have assumed a sophistication which Fox-Rushby comprehensively and comprehensibly outlines. Bech writes from a mental health professional's perspective. He outlines an approach which looks for commonalities between psychiatric classification schemes, the dimensions underlying the many measures for assessing an individual's functional state, and the domains of subjective well-being. Bech describes how this approach, incorporating physical, cognitive, affective, social, economic and ego indicators, has been successfully used in the assessment of clinical improvement during treatment.

Quality of Life Assessment in Cancer

Cancer is a disease with a severe impact on quality of life that occurs with a high frequency and has a pattern of chronicity. In addition the disease often requires highly toxic treatments that are in hand of themselves distressing. A considerable amount of work has been completed on developing measures for the assessment of the functional status and quality of life of cancer patients. However, as Saxena illustrates in his chapter on the quality of life of cancer patients in India, quality of life assessment is as yet a relatively novel concept in India, and little or no work has been done on developing reliable and valid assessments in this setting. Saxena writes about the difficulties of providing adequate health care delivery to this group in a context where early detection is rare, resources for treatment inadequate, and palliative care not yet accepted by oncologists as an effective adjunct or alternative to curative treatments. This is a situation reflected in many developing world countries. Saxena goes on to describe the Indian socio-cultural construction of health and quality of life, and highlights the worldly-spiritual distinction so salient for patients with a terminal illness.

Moinpour describes the work of the Southwest Oncology Group to assess quality of life in cancer clinical trials for new cancer treatments, in particular the work of this group towards developing reliable and valid versions of their measure for use with ethnic minority groups in the USA. With the immigration of large numbers of people into the US, the health care concerns of these groups are an urgent priority. Initiatives such as those taken by Moinpour's group are laudable in highlighting the health needs of these vulnerable groups in the many-sided and complex US health care system. Fallowfield's chapter addresses in a practical way the treatment of breast cancer in health care settings in the UK. She describes the effects of breast cancer on quality of life, the instruments available for assessing the well-being and quality of life of cancer patients, and the applications of quality of life data with this disease group.

Quality of Life Assessment in Specific Populations

WHO has identified five priority groups in international quality of life assessment. The first is patients with chronic diseases, an increasingly large and prominent group of health care users, particularly in industrialised countries where the proportion of elderly persons in the population increases yearly. For example, Skevington describes issues surrounding the assessment of quality of life among those with arthritis, a chronic disease with significant impacts on quality of life, for which treatments in the developed world are increasingly oriented towards palliation and not merely the amclioration of symptoms and disease. Amir describes results from a large-scale controlled clinical trial in which an innovative subjective quality of life assessment is used to assess several treatments for hypertension. Although not reported in the current book, there are many other chronic diseases for which WHO has a range of programmes and activities aimed at effecting improvements in the quality of life of patients with chronic diseases (e.g., HIV/AIDS, epilepsy, diabetes, certain tropical diseases).

A second priority area identified by WHO is the non-professionals, usually family members, who care for patients with chronic diseases and disability – "informal caregivers." Herrman describes a study in which she highlights the considerable burden of caring experienced by informal caregivers, and the needs and circumstances of this important and little recognised group.

A third group identified by WHO as priority groups in quality of life and its assessment are those living in highly stressful situations, such as the mentally ill or elderly living in poorly run large institutions. De Vries and Van Heck describe their work on the development of a quality of life assessment for refugees, thereby underscoring the complex and urgent needs of refugees, of whom there are currently some 14 million in the world.

A fourth group are those who are vulnerable and difficult to assess and treat by nature of their impairment, i.e., those with communication difficulties. This may include people with learning disabilities or those with sight, hearing or speech impairments. A final group are children whose quality of life has traditionally been assessed by proxy, but considerable data have now accumulated suggesting the inadequacy of proxy measures of quality of life. WHO is also developing a methodology for the assessment of the quality of life of children.

The book closes with a chapter from Dazord, which describes her team's innovative work on the development and field testing of a genuinely subjective quality of life assessment for use in therapeutic trials.

J. Orley, W. Kuyken

Acknowledgements

Most of the chapters included in this volume were presented during the course of a meeting on International Quality of Life Assessment in Health Care Settings, held in Paris, France, on July 1 and 2, 1993. The editors wish to express their appreciation to the IPSEN Foundation for hosting and supporting this meeting. In particular we wish to thank Dr. Michel Allard, Scientific and Medical Director of the IPSEN Foundation, for enabling a productive collaboration between the World Health Organization and the IPSEN Foundation in the area of quality of life promotion and assessment. It is also our pleasure to thank Mrs. J. Mervaillie of the IPSEN Foundation for her able assistance in the organization of the meeting, and subsequently in the production of this book, and Mrs. M. L. Gage for her editorial assistance. Thanks are also due to Mrs. L. Kurkcuoglu for the secretarial and administrative support which facilitated much of the planning and organization of the meeting.

Contents

Contributors

Amir M.
Department of Behavioral Sciences, Ben-Gurion University of the Negev, P.O. Box 653, Beer-Sheva 84105, Israel

Bar-on D.
Department of Behavioral Sciences, Ben-Gurion University of the Negev, P.O. Box 653, Beer-Sheva 84105, Israel

Bech P.
Department of Psychiatry, Frederiksborg General Hospital, 48, Dyrehavevej, DK-3400 Hillerod, Denmark

Boissel J.-P.
Unité de Pharmacologie Clinique, 162, Avenue Lacassagne, 69424 Lyon Cedex 03, France

Bullinger M.
Institute for Medical Psychology, Goethestr. 31, D-80336 München, Germany

Cristal N.
Intensive Care Unit – Saroka Medical Center, Ben-Gurion University of the Negev, P.O. Box 653, Beer-Sheva 84105, Israel

Dazord A.
Script-Inserm, Hôpital Saint Jean de Dieu, 290, Route de Vienne, 69008 Lyon, France

De Vries Y.
Department of Psychology, Tilburg University, P.O. Box 90153, 5000 Le Tilburg, The Netherlands

Fallowfield L.
Dept. of Oncology, University College London Medical School, 48, Riding House Street, London W1P 7PL

Fox-Rushby J.A.
Health Policy Unit, London School of Hygiene and Tropical Medicine,
Keppel Street, London WC1E 7 HT, UK

Gerin P.
Script-Inserm, Hôpital Saint Jean de Dieu,
290, Route de Vienne, 69008 Lyon, France

Herrman H.
Department of Psychiatry, St. Vincent's Hospital,
41 Victoria Parade, Fitzroy, Victoria 3065, Australia

Johnson E.S.
Cost and Outcomes Assessment Team,
School of Public Health and Community Medicine,
University of Washington, 146 North Canal Street, Suite 310,
Seattle, WA 98103, USA

Kuyken W.
Division of Mental Health, World Health Organization,
CH-1211 Geneva 27, Switzerland

Martin M.
Cost and Outcomes Assessment Team,
School of Public Health and Community Medicine,
University of Washington, 146 North Canal Street, Suite 310,
Seattle, WA 98103, USA

Moinpour C.M.
Southwest Oncology Group Statistical Center,
Fred Hutchinson Cancer Research Center,
Seattle, WA, USA

Murphy B.
Department of Psychiatry, St. Vincent's Hospital,
41 Victoria Parade, Fitzroy, Victoria 3065, Australia

Orley J.
Division of Mental Health, World Health Organization,
CH-1211 Geneva 27, Switzerland

Patrick, D.L.
Cost and Outcomes Assessment Team,
School of Public Health and Community Medicine,
University of Washington, 146 North Canal Street, Suite 310,
Seattle, WA 98103, USA

Sartorius N.
Division of Mental Health, World Health Organization,
CH-1211 Geneva 27, Switzerland

Saxena S.
Department of Psychiatry, All-India Institute of Medical Sciences,
New Delhi 110029, India

Schofield H.
Department of Psychiatry, St. Vincent's Hospital,
41 Victoria Parade, Fitzroy, Victoria 3065, Australia

Singh B.
Department of Psychiatry, St. Vincent's Hospital,
41 Victoria Parade, Fitzroy, Victoria 3065, Australia

Skevington S.K.
School of Social Sciences, University of Bath,
Bath BA2 7AY, UK

Van Heck G.L.
Department of Psychology, Tilburg University,
P.O. Box 90153, 5000 Le Tilburg, The Netherlands

Wagner T.
Cost and Outcomes Assessment Team,
School of Public Health and Community Medicine,
University of Washington, 146 North Canal Street, Suite 310,
Seattle, WA 98103, USA

Wild D.J.
Cost and Outcomes Assessment Team,
School of Public Health and Community Medicine,
University of Washington, 146 North Canal Street, Suite 310,
Seattle, WA 98103, USA

WHOQOL Group
Division of Mental Health, World Health Organization,
CH-1211 Geneva 27, Switzerland

The Development of Cross-Cultural Quality of Life Assessment Instruments

Translation of Health Status Instruments

N. Sartorius and *W. Kuyken*

Introduction

Methods and instruments to measure the various facets of health status range from ways of calculating mortality and morbidity statistics at regional, national and global levels (e.g., WHO 1991; World Bank 1993) to interview and questionnaire methods for assessing diseases and physical symptoms (e.g., CIDI and SCAN; Pull and Wittchen, 1991), as well as a wealth of instruments for the assessment of impairment, disability, handicap and psychological functioning (see McDowell and Newell 1987; Bowling 1991; WHO 1993a; Walker and Rosser 1993). Most health status measures and psychological tests are used only in the setting in which they were developed. Some are translated into other languages and used without attention to the adaptation that is necessary to ensure their usefulness in another culture or language. A very small number of instruments are produced in equivalent versions in different languages, before assessing the instruments' validity and reliability that are a prerequisite for the use of instruments in a new culture. We shall argue that both properly conducted translation of existing health status instruments and the development of equivalent versions of an instrument in different languages was time consuming and difficult tasks, yet necessities for comparative study.

Equivalent language versions of an instrument make it possible to carry out multicentre research and to meaningfully compare results obtained in different centres. Such research has important benefits, permitting questions to be addressed which would not be possible in single site studies, for example an examination of the effects of different diagnostic practices in two or more countries on health care delivery. In some instances accumulation of cases, particularly when studying rare disorders, is facilitated by gathering data in several settings. Multi-centre collaborative studies can also provide simultaneous multiple replications of a finding, adding considerably to the confidence with which findings can be accepted. The availability of cross-culturally comparable health status measures will also enable comparative international epidemiological studies, thus facilitating the understanding of diseases and the development of treatment methods (Sartorius and Helmchen 1981).

The translation of health status measures to date has commonly failed to acknowledge the complexity of the translation process. Differences exist between cultures in their concepts of health and illness, levels of literacy, reading level, concordance between written and spoken versions of language, taboo subjects,

J. Orley, W. Kuyken (Eds.)
Quality of Life Assessment:
International Perspectives

and social desirability effects. Furthermore, certain features of language, such as idiom, are very difficult to translate, and abound in some health status instruments. Indeed, considerable variability exists in most of these factors even within the same culture. Effective translation methods recognize and address these issues.

In this chapter we shall outline three broad approaches to the translation of health status measures, discuss the conceptual, semantic and technical equivalence which translation should ensure and describe a translation methodology, which can overcome many of the difficulties of translation.

Approaches to Translation

Language is central to the culture in which it is spoken, and cultural factors are often central to the language that is spoken.[1] Language comprises an important and powerful aspect of any national or regional identity. In the many regions of India, for example, language is one of the most characteristic features defining its people (e.g., Kannada, Tamil). Attempts to introduce Hindi as a national language for all the 900 million inhabitants of India have met with singular failure. In Uganda's colonially imposed national boundaries at least 20 languages, and a multitude of dialects, coexist. Since independence English has been maintained as the national language to enable language unity without alienating any of Uganda's many peoples. A person's conception of disease is subject to considerable cultural variation (Kleinman et al. 1978; Kleinman 1980), such that constructs underlying many health status measures cannot be assumed to be culture-free. Thus, illness can only be properly regarded as a normative experience governed by cultural rules (Kleinman et al. 1978). It is easy to see, therefore, how straightforward translation into another language for use in another culture of an instrument which does not take into account cultural and language differences can introduce serious sources of error into results gathered with the target language version of the instrument.

We shall outline four approaches to translation: an ethnocentric approach; a pragmatic approach; an approach incorporating both culture-specific (emic) and culture-general (etic) factors; and an approach which involves an interpretation or re-presentation in the target language.[2]

---

[1] A position commonly referred to as the Sapir-Whorf hypothesis, after two early proponents of this position.

[2] A number of terms are used which require definition at this point. The source language refers to the language that the instrument is *to be translated from*, whilst the target language refers to the language which the instrument *is to be translated into*. Semantic space refers to the denotation and connotation of a word defined in terms of its limits with related concepts. Some words have a broader semantic space (e.g., discomfort), whilst others have a narrower semantic space (e.g., cramp).

The translation of an instrument developed in one culture into the language of another culture, without prior consideration of the appropriateness of the instrument in the target culture, can be regarded as an "ethnocentric approach." This approach makes a number of assumptions. First, that the conceptual dimensions of health covered by the source instrument are transferable to the target culture. Second, that the source and target languages are sufficiently closely related to enable a meaningful translation. Third, that the method of questioning of the source instrument is acceptable in the target culture.

The principal danger of the ethnocentric approach is the distortion in results that results from the use of inappropriate health constructs, which are valid in the source setting but not in the target setting. When the relationship between health constructs in the source and target settings is not explicitly acknowledged and understood, data will be difficult to interpret. This approach was taken with the first translation of the Sickness Impact Profile for use with Spanish-speaking people in the USA. Not surprisingly, the instrument's construct validity in Spanish was found to be poor (Deyo 1984). Although the difference between the Sickness Impact Profile's source and target construct validity may be due to translation difficulties or actual clinical differences in the two groups studied, it is also possible that the same underlying constructs of the impact of disease on daily activities and behaviour cannot be assumed among Mexican Americans. Numerous examples of this approach exist, many with similarly poor results. There are also examples of this approach being used without any acceptable efforts being made to address the construct validity of the target language version.

A second approach involves looking for common ground between the two cultures and measuring and translating only those health constructs found to be common to both cultures. So, for example, with a measure concerned with pain, the aim would be to establish whether the health professionals' and lay understanding of pain was the same in both cultural settings, what extent of semantic space is shared, and what items in the source instrument address this semantic space. This approach can be regarded as pragmatic because the source instrument is adopted for use in the target culture only in so far as it can be regarded to have validity in that culture.

A third approach involves first looking for common ground between cultures in the conceptual basis of an instrument (etic aspects) and translating only the etic items. A further stage involves looking for culture-specific facets of the concept in the target culture, with a view to operationalizing and also measuring them (emic aspects). This approach can be termed an *emic plus etic approach,* i.e., both the concepts specific to the target culture and the concepts found in both cultures are measured. The emic concepts would have to be assessed in separate studies in the two cultures, although these should already be measured in the source instrument.

These three approaches are illustrated in Figure 1, where one can see four possible outcomes. First, the source instrument addresses etic concepts and, by chance or design, no emic facets of this concept exist in the target culture; an ethnocentric approach is warranted. Second, a large degree of overlap exists

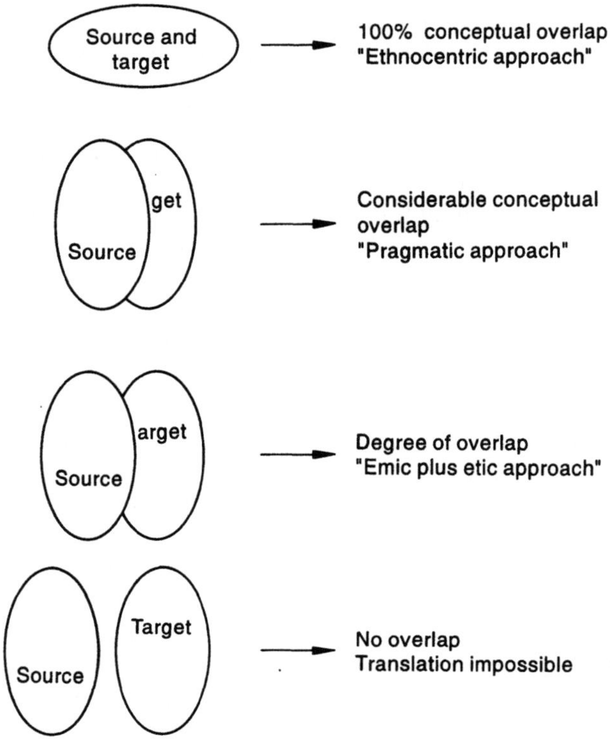

Fig. 1 Approaches to translation of health measures.

in the concept between source and target cultures; a pragmatic approach is warranted. Third, a lesser degree of overlap exists, with significant aspects of the concept being emic to the target culture; an emic plus etic approach is warranted. The final scenario finds no etic features to the concept, and items would have to be developed in each of the cultures in which the studies are conducted.

A fourth approach involves the interpretation of items in the source instrument, for use in the target culture/language. This approach does not involve the presentation of the source instrument in another language but rather a *re-presentation* of the source instrument in another language. A Chinese story illustrates this approach. A Chinese emperor commissioned a tunnel to be dug and asked his counsellors how this might be done most speedily. His counsellors suggested digging from both sides of the mountain simultaneously. The emperor then asked what would happen if the two tunnels did not meet in the middle, to which his counsellors replied, "Then we will have two tunnels." In the same way, it is possible for an instrument to be interpreted in a translation, with the interpretation being guided by the translator's understanding of the target culture. While it is likely that the interpretation approach will be relatively easy to apply in the target culture, it may well happen that the distance from the source language instrument will be so large that the process will result in two similar instruments whose application will not yield comparable data.

Translation and Types of Equivalence

The aim in translating health status measures is to maintain, as far as possible, conceptual, semantic and technical equivalence between the target language and source language versions of the instruments.

Conceptual equivalence refers to the same concepts underlying the questions in an instrument in both source and target languages. For example, one might find that:

For a specific observation a belch is a belch and nepotism is nepotism. But within an inferential framework, a belch is an "insult" or a "compliment," and nepotism is "corruption" or "responsibility"

(Prezeworski and Teune 1970, p. 92).

Koumare et al. (1992), when translating and testing a widely used self-report questionnaire, found that the item "do your hands tremble" was not suitable because in Mali trembling of hands is considered as a sign of a different concept, virility. Some of the items referring to somatic symptoms were difficult to interpret in a setting where many people suffer from diseases likely to cause the same symptoms, and other items seemed to be incomprehensible (e.g., thought interference).

Classical Arabic has a wealth of words associated with the camel (shape, age, condition, equipment), and English probably has equally many associated with the car. If traditional forms of transport are the focus of enquiry, the development of items with conceptual equivalence in the Arabic and English languages poses a considerable challenge. Indeed, an attempt to translate the Nottingham Health Profile into Arabic failed, because Hunt (1986) was unable to find conceptual equivalence for many dimensions underlying the Nottingham Health Profile's items.

Exploring conceptual equivalence can help to define what should be covered by an assessment instrument and indicates ways in which the presence or absence of a phenomenon should be interpreted. Information about conceptual equivalence can be obtained from careful review of relevant cross-cultural work. It is also possible to carry out psychometric analyses to obtain an indication of conceptual equivalence. So, for example, Cattell and his colleagues (1961) applied a personality questionnaire in English and French. A factor analysis of the data showed that the factorial structure remained the same when the test was used in French; there were, however, some items which "changed" their place and "belonged" to different factors in the two languages (Cattell et al. 1961). Thus, the dimensions of personality measured by this test can be said to have conceptual equivalence in the two settings.

Semantic equivalence refers to the denotative and connotative sameness of words. That is to say, what the words indicate or are a sign for (denotation) or what is implied by the words in addition to their emotional meaning (connotation). Denotation of words can be examined on the basis of the definition of words found in dictionaries and relies mainly on linguistic analyses. For example, the two English words "pain" and "ache" denote a semantic difference which does not exist in Croatian. Thus, an English pain measure with two items, one addressing pain and the other addressing ache, would lose one item if translated into Croatian. Similarly, the term often used in English measures, "problems with your nerves," cannot be translated literally into Dutch and would be "geestelijke problemen" (mental problems). In these cases, the semantic space surrounding the source language item needs to be examined, and items need to be identified which address that same space in the target language.

Connotation of words can be studied using results of anthropological analyses and techniques such as Osgood's semantic differential (1952) and Kelly's repertory grid (1955).

The semantic equivalence of words can also be studied by comparison of their semantic spaces. Synonyms of a word describe the semantic space which the word occupies, an equivalent word in another language occupies a similar semantic space. The process of examining semantic space can be time consuming and is not usually carried out for all the terms which are used in a measure. In the following question addressing an individual's sense of self-efficacy, "How often do you avoid doing things because you might fail?," for example,[3] it is likely that the word "avoid" would be a candidate for such an examination. This would proceed as follows:

AVOID has in a medium-size dictionary the following corresponding words in French (for the different situations in which it is used):
éviter
échapper
esquiver
se soustraire
frauder
fuir
se dispenser.

The word *éviter* is, according to the dictionary, closest to the act of avoiding a person or a situation. Its meanings can be translated into English by:
avoid
dodge
steer clear of

[3] English and French semantic equivalence was selected for this example to facilitate matters for readers who are not conversant with more distant languages.

duck
evade
prevent.

The translation of the other words describing *avoid* in French can be rendered into English by:

échapper –	escape, get away from, elude
esquiver –	sidestep, dodge
se soustraire –	shirk, get out
frauder –	shirk, cheat, elude
fuir –	fly, run away
se dispenser –	liberate, shirk, get rid of.

The translation of the other words describing *éviter* in French can be rendered in English by:

dodge –	mouvement de côté, esquiver, détour
steer clear of –	se tenir à l'écart, éviter, fuir, s'abstenir
duck –	esquiver un coup
evade –	esquiver, éviter, échapper, se dérober, se soustraire, contourner, frauder
prevent –	empêcher, éviter.

A comparison is now possible between the two English and two French sets of near-synonyms. It shows that the word "éviter," by its synonyms, "matches" the word "avoid" in the sense defined by the context of the question. There are certain terms (such as "se dérober," "contourner," "empêcher") which do not have an exact correspondent term in the English series, and it is also probable that the translation of avoid by "éviter" in the sentence cited is correct, but that the word "éviter" would thus not necessarily have to be translated by "avoid" if the original were in French and the target language were English.

The choice of synonyms usually employed for a word depends on the linguistic context. In the spoken language some of the synonyms will appear predominantly in a particular context, determined by the social class of the speakers, their closeness and shared memories and traditions. In professional groups belonging to the same discipline, the choice of synonyms will also be firmly determined. Deviation from the customary choice of synonyms can lead to misunderstanding and emotional tension.

Furthermore, translations which seem identical on consideration of the back-translation of the target instrument can contain implicit connotations which lie beyond a strict interpretation of the words. For example the item "I feel fed up" in UK English means dejected, despondent, and weary; whilst in USA English it has a more angry, frustrated and irascible connotation[4].

[4] We take the position that items cannot be assumed to have conceptual or semantic equivalence across major anglophone centres: e.g., Australia, Canada, Uganda, UK and USA. UK English words/terms such as "getting off to sleep" (going to sleep), "perhaps" (maybe), "recreation" (leisure) and even "such as" (for example) would be regarded as "foreign" in a health measure in North America.

A further example is provided by the translation of the item "How well are you able to carry out your daily activities (for example washing, dressing and preparing food)?" into the Indian languages of Hindi and Tamil. The translators interpreted the word "washing" to refer to clothes, not bathing, and even the back-translation failed to flag this different interpretation. Only the types of linguistic analyses outlined above would identify such semantic incongruities in the two language versions.

Technical equivalence refers to two separate but overlapping issues: first, the equivalence of technical features of language and their relationship to the socio-cultural context; and second, the feasibility of the nature and mode of questioning of the instrument in both source and target culture.

In relation to the technical features of language, equivalence of features of language such as grammar and syntax should be maintainable. In Vietnamese, for example, and in some other languages, there is no conditional tense. It is therefore difficult to formulate questions illustrated by examples to clarify the interviewer's intent. Similarly, technical equivalence also applies to language complexity, question length and acceptable levels of abstraction in questions. In a Puerto Rican Spanish translation of the Diagnostic Interview Schedule for Children, several items were found to be long and difficult to understand and could be shortened or simplified without loss of meaning in the Spanish version (Bravo et al. 1993). The Hebrew language is thought to be more economical than English; conversely Latin languages are somewhat less economical than English, i.e., translations may sometimes need fewer or more words than the source instrument to convey the same meaning.

An example of the relationship of language to its socio-cultural context is illustrated by a study in Uganda by Orley and Wing (1979). In England it is acceptable to ask a question such as "What about your interests, have they changed at all,?" which the subject may answer by describing a loss of interest if this was the case. In Uganda, Orley and Wing (1979) found it impossible to obtain more than a vague negative answer to this question and had to change the form of enquiry to a dual exploration of a loss and an increase of interests. In some cultures, direct questioning about certain issues (e.g., sexual functioning, financial status, use of alcohol) is not possible for reasons of form and etiquette, and a round-about manner of investigation is necessary. For example in the cultural context of Northern India, the question "How would you rate your ability to remember things?" is construed as being unacceptable and patronizing.

Technical equivalence also refers to the form of questioning of the instrument, which assumes familiarity among respondents with a particular form of enquiry. It is easy for the researcher/interviewer to lose sight of the fact that an interview and administered questionnaire are essentially transactions between two strangers which involve personal questions and may therefore be highly uncomfortable in certain settings.

High levels of illiteracy in some countries mean that interviewer-assisted or interviewer-administered forms of a measure need to be used, raising questions about technical equivalence. If an interviewer-administered form of a questionnaire is used which was a self-administered questionnaire in its source language, technical equivalence cannot be assumed. Multi-trait, multi-method approaches should be used to establish the correspondence between these different forms of the instrument. Comparisons should be carried out at each level: comparing results obtained with different forms of the instrument within each culture, as well as comparing results obtained with the same form of the instrument in different cultures.

Achieving technical equivalence is particularly difficult in the case of fully standardized instruments which have to be used in exactly the same manner by all the interviewers. In semi-standardized interviews, in which the meaning of an item is made clear to the investigator, this difficulty can be overcome by using ways of contextualising the issues in a culturally appropriate way. Clearly, the onus of ensuring cross-cultural technical comparability is then placed on the training of investigators which has to impart full understanding of the nature of the rating that is required in a particular area.

Achieving semantic, conceptual and technical equivalence of standardized and semi-standardized instruments is more complex when the instrument is to be used in more than two languages. The method most frequently used to achieve equivalence among the different language versions is to compare each version with the source version, assuming that the two versions which are equivalent to a third will also be equivalent between themselves. This is not necessarily the case. In a WHO study to develop a Quality of Life assessment (WHO 1993; WHOQOL Group 1993), the translations of the pilot instrument were first compared with the working language version, English, but then further language comparisons were made between centres (e.g., French and Dutch; American English and French).

These three types of equivalence, conceptual, semantic and technical, should be explicitly addressed in the translation process to ensure equivalence of the source and target language versions of the health measure.

Recommended Procedure for Translation of Health Measures

WHO has accrued considerable experience in translating health measurements. This has facilitated the development of a translation methodology which has significant advantages over the forward-translation and the translation-back-translation methodologies. The steps outlined below describe a sequence which has been used successfully in a number if studies. It is clear that variations of the method may well be necessary, and indeed desirable, in certain situations.

Preparation for Translation

In the translation of existing health status instruments a thorough examination of the rationale for, and feasibility of, translation is an important first step. The proposed uses of the instrument in the target culture should be consistent with the stated uses of the source instrument. An exploration of appropriate existing instruments in the target culture with adequate psychometric properties of validity and reliability should be carried out. If there are none available, a rationale for the translation should be stated. The rationale should address the comparability of the dimensions of the source instrument (e.g., functional status, or quality of life) in the two cultures. One way of exploring the appropriateness of the instrument's dimensions in the target culture is to use the operational definitions from the source instrument and test these in a series of focus groups with health care users and health care professionals in the target culture. Focus group participants are presented with the dimensions covered by the instrument and guided towards a discussion of their appropriateness in the target culture. The question of whether any important facets of the construct are missing should be explicitly addressed in the focus groups.

These data should then be used to assess the suitability of the instrument for translation and the possibility of any additional facets of the construct being added (see Figure 1). This should, wherever possible, be done in consultation with the instrument authors to avoid "the wheel being reinvented"; it is possible that several constructs were not addressed in the source instrument for good reasons[5]. Any new facets should then be operationalized, with a view to subsequent writing of these items[6].

[5] Approval for translation should anyway be sought from the instrument authors and/or copyright holders. This will help avoid the undesirable situation where a number of unauthorised translated versions with differing psychometric properties exist in a given language. International guidelines on copyright state that the author "has the exclusive right to (a) make a translation, (b) publish a translation, (c) authorise the making of a translation, and (d) authorise the publication of a translation" (Stewart and Sandison 1989, p. 162).

[6] This may appear a lot of work but will avoid the enormous investment involved in translating and testing an instrument, only to find it performs poorly in the target language. For example, in the translation of an English family dynamics measure into Finnish, failure to carry out this phase resulted in very low internal consistency on two of the scales (White and Elander 1992). Numerous other examples exist in the literature, and many more, one can assume, which were never published.

The Translation Process

The following individuals will need to assist in the translation process:

1) **A bilingual panel** (three to six individuals)
The group should consist of individuals skilled in interviewing and assessment, as well as clinicians and behavioural scientists, particularly anthropologists. The group will examine the overall form of the instrument and learn how to apply it. A skilled user of the instrument would ideally demonstrate its use and discuss its features with the bilingual group.
2) **Monolingual individuals** (at least four) who will be able to comment in an articulate way on the translated document. The monolingual group should be representative of the people who are likely to use the instrument in the target culture and of those who will be subjects in the proposed studies.
3) **Three translators.**

PHASES OF TRANSLATION PROCESS

I. PREPARATION FOR TRANSLATION

Identification of candidate instrument

Approval/copyright for translation

Examination of candidate instrument's appropriateness
(etic aspects of candidate instrument)

Creation of bilingual panel

Identification and operationalization of emic constructs

II. TRANSLATION PROCESS

Translation by 2 translators working together

Writing of emic items

Monolingual review

Bilingual review

Linguistic analyses

Back-translation by independent translator

Iteration, if needed

III. QUALITY CONTROL MEASURES

Review by bilingual panel

Iteration, if needed

IV. RELIABILITY AND VALIDITY STUDIES

Review by bilingual panel

Fig. 2. Translation methodology for health status measures[7]

---

[7] This figure is based on a figure in Sartorius (1994) outlining the different approaches required for the translation of standardised and semi-standardised health status instruments.

The translation process has a number of steps. The source instrument is translated into the target language by two translators, who consult one another in the course of their work. These translators should have a clear and detailed understanding of the instrument and the population who will use the instrument. This will increase the likelihood both that the instrument is translated appropriately and that the language levels used in the translated document match closely the language usage of the target group.

The bilingual panel then reviews the translation, looking for any inconsistencies between the source language version and the translated document, and discussing and resolving issues related to the maintenance of the integrity of the source instrument in terms of conceptual, semantic and technical equivalence.

A group of monolinguals, unfamiliar with the instrument, and representative of the population for whom the instrument is intended, then "tests" the document by reading through it, looking for aspects of the translation which are not clearly comprehensible or are ambiguous in the target language. The presentation of the instrument to monolinguals is of considerable importance because they rely only on the text in the target language and have no prior idea of the concepts the item was designed to address, nor the form or content of the item in the source language. Monolingual review can be done in a focus group situation, where focus group participants arrive having read through the instrument and discuss the instrument in session. This would involve detailed discussion of the instrument's instructions, items and response scales. Ideally such monolingual focus groups would be moderated by a member of the bilingual panel.

The bilingual group then considers the comments of the monolingual group and, wherever these accurately reflect the source document, incorporates them into the translated document. It is at this stage that the linguistic analyses outlined above can be usefully done. This group should also ensure that the document is grammatically correct in the target language.

The translated document is then back-translated to the original language. By another translator who should be briefed about his/her place in the translation methodology being used and told that s/he is translating a measure concerned with health. This ensures the translator's work is appropriate to the methodology without introducing bias into the process.

Quality Control Measures

An ideal way of ensuring equivalence is for the instrument to be applied to bilingual respondents successively in the two language versions. The space between administration should be short enough to ensure no change in health status has occurred but long enough to ensure that respondents do not simply recall what they responded before. Half the respondents should complete the source language version first, the other half should complete the target language version first. Identical scores for the two language versions would indicate equivalence has been achieved. However, this would present the difficulty of finding sufficient bilingual respondents, perhaps even within disease groups. Alternative ways of establishing equivalence include bilingual committee review, checking of terms through the target check method (Sartorius 1979) and textual analyses in which the equivalence of words is judged by the likelihood of using them in the same context in the two languages. In addition bilingual raters can independently rate the quality of the translation along a number of dimensions and identify consistent differences between source and target versions of the instrument. If significant differences are apparent, further bilingual review and translation/back-translation need to be done until a successful transfer of meaning is achieved.

Item and Response Scale Management

Item Management

In the translation of health status measures, items may need to be handled in one of at least three ways: a complete set of items may need to be written for subsequent translation into one or more languages; existing items may need to be modified; and additional items may need to be devised for an existing set of items.

When instruments are developed simultaneously in several cultures, it is important to ensure that items are amenable to translation. A prerequisite in any item writing is clear and concise definitions of the concepts which items should address. A complete conceptual definition should ideally consist of: 1) a description of the concept; 2) a description of various indicators or dimensions along which a rating can be made for that concept; 3) a listing of some example situations or conditions that might significantly affect that concept, at various levels of intensity. Brislin and his colleagues have suggested a number of guidelines for writing translatable items (Brislin et al. 1973; Brislin 1986). Questions should be phrased in the active voice, be short and concise, provide context, repeat nouns rather than use pronouns, and use specifics rather than generalities. Questions should avoid metaphors or colloquialisms, the subjunctive, more than one verb per question, and words which are vague (e.g., probably, sometimes). When an instrument is developed without any explicit plan for subsequent translation, understandably these latter guidelines are rarely followed, and instruments result which are linguistically more complex and ethnocentric. White and Elander (1992) describe the translation of an English instrument assessing family dynamics into several Nordic languages. English language colloquialisms such as "I feel blue," "I am a loner," and "I get stuck with all the bad jobs," proved difficult to translate and needed a series of iterative back-translations to achieve equivalence.

If a source item does not have a readily available target language equivalent, then items may have to be modified or deleted. In the modification of items, careful attention should be paid to maintaining technical consistency in items within the instrument. In relation to response scales, the magnitude of the response to the target question should be the same as the magnitude of the response of an identical respondent in the source language. In subsequent quality control tests, and reliability and validity studies, modified items should be scrutinized carefully. Where items are added, as with the emic plus etic approach outlined above, items obviously do not need to meet the same criteria as for translatable items. Instead, they should follow the same form as the core items and be clearly comprehensible. Within an emic plus etic approach to translation, any additional items in the target language instrument can be incorporated into the translation process by including them among the items which are considered in monolingual and subsequent bilingual review (see Fig. 2).

Response Scale Management

To ensure international comparability of health status instruments, derivation of equivalent or comparable response scales is critical. Translation of response scales is fraught with difficulty. Words which make good response scale descriptors in one language may not translate into good descriptors in another language. Similarly changes in shade of meaning turn out to be more marked following data collection than was originally supposed in the translation process. Although endpoints such as "never" and "always" are relatively universal, shades of meaning between endpoints (e.g., "sometimes") are more ambiguous, difficult to translate, and subject to cultural variation in their interpretation. In the WHO project to develop an international Quality of Life assessment (the WHOQOL) a methodology was used to derive equivalent response scales in each language (this methodology is described in the chapter by the WHOQOL Group in this volume). An alternative method for ensuring the equivalence of response scales is to prepare a series of vignettes with a full range of health status. These are then translated into the target language(s). Independent health personnel then rate each vignette on where it would score on a response scale. The response scale language version ratings are then compared. Consistently different ratings for given points on the response scales would suggest that response scales are not equivalent.

Following translation, the measure should be subjected to reliability and validity studies in the target culture. The following psychometric properties of the translated instrument should be assessed: test-retest reliability, internal consistency, responsiveness to change and construct validation, specifically with regard to convergent, discriminant and predictive validity. This latter is a crucial process and would preferably be over several samples.

Summary and Conclusion

The development of equivalent versions of health status instruments which will be used in comparative (cross-cultural) studies is an important part of preparation for multi-centre research. The methods for the translation of health status instruments are well developed and can ensure conceptual, semantic and technical equivalence between the versions of an instrument in different languages. Translation of health status measures should use a pragmatic approach that identifies aspects of health that are common to both cultures, as well as any features of health which are specific to the settings which are being studied. The steps which are necessary to arrive at equivalent translations would ideally involve focus group work, a bilingual review panel, testing of the translation by monolinguals and a series of quality control measures.

References

Bowling A (1991) Measuring health: a review of quality of life measurement scales. Philadelphia, Open University Press

Bravo M, Woodbury-Farina, Canino GJ, Rubio-Stipec M (1993) The Spanish translation and cultural adaptation of the Diagnostic Interview Schedule for Children (DISC) in Puerto Rico. Culture Med Psychiat 17:329–344

Brislin RW (1986) The wording and translation of research instruments. In: Lonner WJ, Berry JW (eds) Field methods in cross-cultural research. Beverley Hills, CA, Sage Publications

Brislin RW, Lonner WJ, Thorndike RM (1973) Cross-cultural research methods. New York, Wiley

Cattell R, Pichot P, Rennes P (1961) Constance interculturelle des facteurs de personnalité mesurée par le test 16 PF. Comparison franco-américaine. Rev Psychol Appliquée 11:165–196

Deyo R (1984) Pitfalls in measuring the health status of Mexican Americans: Comparative validity of the English and Spanish Sickness Impact Profile. Am J Public Health 74:569–573

Hunt SM (1986) Cross-cultural issues in the use of socio-medical indicators. Health Pol 6:149–158

Kelly GA (1955) A theory of personality. New York, Norton and Co

Kleinman A (1980) Patients and healers in the context of culture. Berkeley, University of California Press

Kleinman A, Eisenberg L, Good B (1978) Culture, illness and care: Clinical lessons from anthropologic and cross-cultural research. Ann Internal Med 88:251–258

Koumare B, Diaoure R, Miguel-Garcia E (1992) Défintion d'un instrument de dépistage des troubles psychiques. Psychopathol Afric 24:229–242

McDowell I, Newell C (1987) Measuring health: a guide to rating scales and questionnaires. New York, Oxford University Press

Orley J, Wing JK (1979) Psychiatric disorders in two African villages. Arch Gen Psychiat 36:513–520

Osgood CE (1952) The nature and measurement of meaning. Psychol Bull 49:197–237

Prezeworski A, Teune H (1970) The logic of comparative social enquiry. New York, Wiley

Pull CB, Wittchen H-U (1991) CIDI, SCAN and IPDE: Structured diagnostic interviews for ICD-10 and DSM-III-R. Eur Psychiat 47:589–593

Sartorius N (1979) Cross-cultural psychiatry. In: Kisker KP, Meyer JE, Müller C, Strömgren E (eds) Psychiatrie der Gegenwart, Bd. I/1, Second Edition. Berlin: Springer-Verlag
Sartorius N (1994) SCAN Translation. In: Wing J, Sartorius N, Üstün TB (eds) Diagnosis and clinical measurements in psychiatry: a reference manual for the SCAN system. London, Cambridge University Press
Sartorius N, Helmchen H (1981) Aims and implementation of multi-centre studies. Modern Problems Pharmacopsychiat 16, 1–8
Stewart SM, Sandison H (1989) International copyright and neighbouring rights. London, Butterworths
Walker SR, Rosser RM (eds) (1993) Quality of life assessment: key Issues in the 1990's. Lancaster, UK, Kluwer Academic Publishers
White M, Elander G (1992) Translation of an instrument: The US-Nordic family dynamics nursing research project. Scand J Caring Sci 6:161–164
World Bank (1993) World development report: investing in health. New York, Oxford University Press
World Health Organization (1991) World Health Statistics Annual. Geneva, WHO
World Health Organization (1993a) WHOQOL Study Protocol. WHO (MNH/PSF/93.9)
World Health Organization (1993b) Catalogue of assessment instruments used in the studies coordinated by the WHO Mental Health Programme. Geneva, WHO (WHO/MNH/92.5)
The WHOQOL Group (1993) Study protocol for the World Health Organization project to develop a quality of life assessment instrument (WHOQOL). Quality Life Res 2:153–159

Cross-Cultural Validation of Quality of Life Measures

D.L. Patrick, D.J. Wild, E.S. Johnson, T.H. Wagner and *M.A. Martin*

Summary

Demand is increasing for quality of life measures available for cross-national comparison or aggregation of data across cultures. It is important, therefore, to ensure that an instrument developed in one culture is valid in another. To illustrate an approach to validation, we present a case study of the development of a cross-cultural, quality of life measure specific to genital herpes. The achievement of cross-cultural comparability requires attention to the following issues: 1) the content of the questionnaire and its conceptual basis, 2) the method of translation, and 3) the testing and comparison of reliability, validity, responsiveness, and effect size within each country or culture. In addition to methodological problems, practical considerations include communication difficulties among investigators and the additional expenses involved. Recruiting comparable samples of persons in different countries is also a major challenge to cross-cultural validation. Overcoming these problems will require a higher level of cooperation and coordination between countries. Such studies are lengthy and expensive, requiring commitment of resources and time for the development of valid, reliable, and responsive cross-cultural quality of life measures.

Introduction and Rationale

Demand is increasing throughout the world for quality of life measures that are available in several languages and are appropriate for use in different cultures. This rising demand is due in part to the development of global perspectives on health and health care. Clinical trials are increasingly international, leading to the need to aggregate data across sample populations from different countries. Provision and regulation of health, though still primarily a national responsibility, are affected by transnational agreements on provider licensing and certification, standards of care, and applications of medical technology. The approval process and market for treatments, particularly pharmaceuticals, are becoming more international. This global perspective has prompted development of quality of life measures in which data can be aggregated across different cultures.

J. Orley, W. Kuyken (Eds.)
Quality of Life Assessment:
International Perspectives

Interest in cross-cultural, quality of life measures is furthered by the desire to strengthen causal inference in the evaluation of treatments. As diagnostic criteria become more international, treatment is becoming more standardized in different cultures, thus prompting attempts to compare outcomes of treatment in different cultural settings, particularly using randomized clinical trials. Causal inference and external validity may be strengthened if the same effect is found cross-culturally. Finally, there is a growing interest in comparing different geographical regions, different social and physical environments, and different populations to identify optimal social and health policies, to monitor trends, and to make political claims.

The move toward development of cross-culturally applied measures of quality of life is tempered by the recognition that wide differences exist in the cultural notions of health and illness and in how different populations react to what is presumably the same biological condition. As cultural anthropologists demonstrate repeatedly, a person's conception of what constitutes "disease" or "health" can depend on his or her cultural traditions, language, and group mores as well as more individual characteristics such as age, educational level and income (Fabrega 1974; Kleinman et al. 1978). Consequently, comparisons cannot be made without considering the cultural content of measures. The cross-cultural content of measures, the cultural meaning of different domains, the translation of measures from one language to another, and the cross-cultural testing of measurement properties are important considerations in assessing quality of life.

This paper addresses important issues in cross-cultural research on the validation of quality of life measures. The psychometric or measurement properties of these measures are defined and methods for evaluating these properties in international studies are suggested. The feasibility of such validation is addressed through consideration of the barriers to and opportunities for international cooperation in the development and testing of quality of life measures. A case example of the cross-cultural development of a measure of quality of life specific to genital herpes is used as well as other examples from the literature. Finally, important issues for future cross-cultural research on quality of life assessments are identified.

Issues in Cross-Cultural Research

To the extent that functional status – defined as activities such as walking, sleeping, eating, and working – is found in every culture, it seems reasonable that an instrument assessing function could produce valid cross-cultural results. There appears to be a core set of specific behaviors that transfer readily between cultures. Symptoms may also be described similarly in different cultures. Subjective reactions to symptoms and health conditions – that is, the value assigned to health and living conditions, the relative importance of different states, standards of behavior, and the meaning of different health states

– may show more cultural variation. These subjective perceptions, particularly values and preferences for health, define quality of life (Patrick and Erickson 1993; WHOQOL Group 1993). The extent to which functional status and broader quality of life domains have universal definitions and meaning across cultures is both a theoretical and empirical question.

Cross-cultural comparability also seems plausible to the extent that biology and its consequences are something all persons tend to share, with some exceptions. Similarly, because the social roles of parent, worker and student are comparable, they provide opportunities for evaluating function cross-culturally. However, the inclusion of more culturally specific domains (or the necessary exclusion of others) as well as variation in the natural history of disease, are barriers to the design of valid, cross-cultural instruments. It may be unclear if differences between cultures for quality of life scores should be attributed to variation in the biological response, the cultural setting, the psychosocial constructs used in measurement, or the measurement process itself.

What is meant by cross-cultural? For many parts of the world, cross-cultural cannot be equated with cross-national, because of the ethnic diversity that exists within national boundaries. The assumption of cultural comparability in measures derived from a single sample in a country, therefore, may be invalid. In practice, however, the early development of a measure may begin with a single sample representing a nation, with extensions to different groups at a later date. It is one thing to claim cross-cultural validity for an instrument that has been tested in Europe and the United States; it is quite another to extend this claim to African or Asian cultures. How many cultures – and what scope of cultural variation – are necessary to test the cross-cultural validity of a quality of life instrument? At a minimum it seems that the unqualified use of the phrase "cross-culturally valid" is not particularly informative.

The development of a standard quality of life measure that is applicable and acceptable in many countries requires a different approach to methodological and theoretical issues than is usually taken within the national context. Cultural and linguistic differences can have a significant effect on the way individuals perceive their experiences of health and illness (Hunt 1993).

A Case Study: Genital Herpes and Quality of Life

Genital herpes is caused by Herpes Simplex Virus Type II. It is believed to be one of the most widespread sexually transmitted viral diseases in the world. More than 40 million Americans between the ages of 15 and 74 carry the virus that causes genital herpes, although most will never become symptomatic (Wellcome Dialog 1992). Typically genital herpes is characterized by distinct phases. Two to ten days after infection the individual will experience symptoms including pain when urinating; pain in the buttocks, legs or vaginal area; a feeling of pressure in the genital area, a discharge from the vagina or urethra, or tender lymph nodes. Additional symptoms are those often experienced in any viral infection: fever, chills, muscle aches, lethargy, and headaches. One or more painful blisters will develop, which then crust over and heal. It is not uncommon, however, to have a first time infection without any noticeable symptoms or with minimal discomfort. After the blister(s) has/have disappeared, the virus will travel to the base of an affected nerve supplying the area and become dormant. Generally, the infected individual will have a recurrent outbreak within three to six months of the first outbreak, though these subsequent outbreaks are usually not as severe. For those who have recurrent outbreaks, herpes recurs on average four to six times a year. After a number of years, however, outbreaks tend to become less frequent and less severe. Most people are unable to pinpoint what triggers a herpes outbreak, because outbreaks tend to occur randomly. However, some people identify lack of sleep, poor diet, stress, and menstruation as factors. At this time there is no cure for genital herpes. However, antiviral medications, such as acyclovir, actually stop the virus from replicating. Antivirals can be used for episodic treatment or for suppressive therapy in those with severe or frequent outbreaks. Other treatments, such as the use of L-lysine, remain largely unsubstantiated to date (Corey 1989).

Genital herpes is of significant public health importance, and it has an obvious impact on the quality of life of those infected with the virus. However, no quality of life instrument currently exists for assessing the impact or treatment of genital herpes. The University of Washington is participating in a project to develop such an instrument that is valid cross-culturally. Other countries involved in the project include Denmark, France, Germany, Italy, Spain, and the United Kingdom. Draft items for the instrument were initially developed in the United Kingdom. These items were then translated for use in validation studies in the other countries. In this process, additional items were generated and other items deleted. The instrument has been field tested for respondent acceptance, burden, and cognition. It is currently being assessed for reliability, validity, and responsiveness.

Translation Prior to Validation

Conceptual equivalence means whether the same concept exists in another culture. Semantic equivalence refers to whether the same expression exists in another language or culture. Where conceptual and semantic equivalence are both present, the items in a cross-cultural measure are identical across languages. If the concept exists but not the expression, then the solution is to change the expression in the new language. If the expression exists but not the concept, then the item is culturally specific. If neither the concept nor the expression is present, then it is impossible to render the item into the other language (Hunt 1993).

The difference between conceptual and semantic equivalence can be illustrated using the herpes example. Conceptual equivalence was difficult to achieve for the concept of "dating" in the North American culture. The American ritual of "dating" as a way of initiating intimate relationships does not exist in the same way in some European countries. To ensure cross-cultural validity, quality of life issues in the herpes instrument dealing with relationships are worded as "personal relationships" with a parenthetical "intimate" in the American version. This represents the sort of trade-off necessary in developing cross-cultural instruments: some specificity and clarity is sacrificed in order that the more general domain is assessed for each culture.

Semantic equivalence is more a matter of translation for use in other cultures. Before the validity of an existing quality of life measure can be assessed, instruments created in one language must be translated for use in other cultures. Translations are being conducted with varying degrees of care and sensitivity to the linguistic, technical, and cultural issues involved. Translations that are apparently identical often conceal differences in the meaning of the constructs. In cross-cultural research, translation may occur without consideration of cross-cultural equivalence. Furthermore, translation alone might mean that additional issues are not covered in the instrument, and irrelevant issues are addressed. Protocols and techniques for obtaining an accurate and culturally valid second language translation of instruments are available for use (Del Greco et al. 1987). Four major phases should occur in the translation process: preliminary translation, evaluation of preliminary translations, ascertainment of cross-language equivalence, and assessment of validity, reliability, and responsiveness.

Even adapting a British measure for use in America requires a translation process. For example, the British English version of the draft herpes instrument used the expression "passing water" which is a term not used in common American English, and it was necessary to change this to "urination," a more technical term but one in common usage. Furthermore, the term "attack" when referring to herpes is in common usage in British English, and "outbreak" is more often used in American English. Although subtle, these issues are important to consider prior to the validation process.

The Validation Process: Psychometric Testing

It cannot be assumed that a questionnaire, however extensively tested in the originating country, will be valid and reliable once it has been translated. No instrument for the assessment of psychological states of subjective perceptions is culture-free. In each instance the validity and other metric characteristics of the instrument must be assessed in the culture of application. Important components of psychometric testing in cross-cultural quality of life studies include reliability, validity, responsiveness, and effect size interpretation.

Reliability

Reliability is a generic term that refers to stability and equivalence of repeated measures of the same concept. Reliability coefficients estimate the proportion of observed variation in a score that can be considered true as opposed to random error (Nunnally 1978). *Internal consistency reliability* is the correlation among items in an instrument. Coefficient "alpha" is used to estimate the degree of equivalence between responses to sets of items or questions tapping the same concept. Coefficient alpha will be higher the more items that are included in the measure of a particular concept or domain, and the higher the average correlation between responses to all possible combination of items in the domain.

For discriminating between persons in cross-sectional studies, internal consistency reliability is important. For longitudinal investigations where change over time is assessed, reproducibility, stability, and responsiveness are important to distinguish between those who remain stable and those who experience change. In cross-cultural validation studies, assessing the internal consistency of a question is straightforward. Coefficient alpha can be calculated on all component domains of the instrument. The higher the coefficient, the better the internal consistency of the measure. An acceptable level of alpha for quality of life measures has been defined as 0.70 or above (Stewart and Ware 1992). In most cases this level will be relatively easy to achieve if multiple items are generated and tested for each quality of life domain.

Reproducibility or test-retest reliability refers to the correlation between responses to the same items administered to the same respondents at different times. If something is highly variable by nature, it is difficult to observe whether differences in repeated measures are caused by a chance in the observed phenomenon or by non-reproducible observations. With quality of life measures, reproducibility is preferably measured using the interclass correlation coefficient, which corrects for agreement that would be expected simply by chance (Deyo et al. 1991).

Reproducibility can be tested in each cross-cultural setting by administering the quality of life measure at an interval long enough to avoid recall of previous answers and test learning, but short enough that the actual states or perceptions are likely to remain the same. Reproducibility of the herpes-specific quality of life measure is being assessed by the administration of the instrument at base line and again two weeks later. Clinical status of participants will be assessed at both times to control for possible differences in herpes symptoms. For the questionnaire as a whole, the interclass correlation coefficient will be used to assess the degree of reliability. A correlation of 0.70 will be considered necessary to claim a reproducible instrument.

Validity

Measurement methodologies are widely available for estimating the internal consistency and reproducibility of quality of life measures. Techniques for assessing validity are more limited. Validity is a more emotionally charged term than reliability, because conceptions vary widely about how investigators might be led astray in drawing conclusions from the data. The three most common approaches to assessing validity are reviewed, with a discussion about their applicability to the herpes measure.

Content validity refers to whether a particular measure adequately represents the domain or universe of content it is supposed to measure. Ware (1987) recommends including physical, mental, social, and perceptual health as a minimum standard for content in comprehensive generic measures of health-related quality of life. Content validity can be assessed using other methods. For example, Aday (1990) suggests reviewing the literature and ensuring that at least one item is represented on the questionnaire for each domain identified.

The content validity of the herpes-specific instrument is based on the use of the needs-based model and ethnographic interviews with persons with genital herpes and from two independent reviews of the literature. Hunt and McKenna (1992) developed the "needs-based approach" as a theoretical model to ensure content validity during the development phase of a quality of life measure. In this model, both conceptual and semantic equivalence are required before an item can be included in a cross-cultural instrument. This approach differs greatly in that it does not involve translation of an existing instrument developed in only one country; rather, it involves the concurrent development of an instrument that is intended for cross-cultural application from its inception. The work began in relation to a new measure in quality of life and depression.

Development of the herpes-specific instrument has proceeded using the needs-based approach in that the instrument was developed simultaneously in each country rather than being developed completely in one and translated for use in other countries. *Ethnographic interviews* are used in the needs-based approach for item generation and to assess content validity of an instrument. This technique was used for the herpes-specific instrument in the United Kingdom. Individual interviews were used to generate items for the instrument. In each country, individual interviews were held to assess the content validity of the instrument.

In the United States, a cognitive debriefing exercise was used during the ethnographic interview, giving a structure to the interview and ensuring that the instrument was thoroughly evaluated. Techniques of cognitive debriefing or cognitive interviewing include concurrent think aloud responses to items, retrospective think aloud, focused interviews, and paraphrasing (Jobe and Mingay 1989). In the development of the herpes-specific instrument, people with herpes were asked to complete a draft of the questionnaire, describe important issues they felt were not addressed, and identify any problems in the wording of the items. Each item was then evaluated individually for its clarity, relevance, and wording. Comments from each country were compiled and integrated into the instrument in the United Kingdom. This process eventually resulted in items being added and dropped and existing items being reworded.

Another method for ensuring content validity involves *factor analysis*. Factor analysis can serve many purposes, including determining the latent variable structure underlying a set of items, providing a means of explaining variation among many original variables, and defining the substantive content or meaning of the factors (DeVellis 1991). If a set of items tested in different languages and cultures demonstrate a similar factor structure, this similarity is an indication of shared core meaning and organization of meaning for the items under investigation. Countries can be compared on the items that contribute to the shared content as well as those that do not. Some items may be country- or culture-specific. For example, similarity of the factor structure in British and French populations was accepted as evidence of validity for a quality of life scale for older adults (Guinot and Wesnes 1985). A lack of comparable factor structure has also been used to determine a lack of validity in a quality of life study regarding community satisfaction. Although the notion of community appears to have been understood by both British and American participants, the meaning of the items differed substantially (Bardo and Hughey 1984).

Although factor analysis has been used by investigators to suggest that an instrument is cross-culturally valid because the underlying "factor structure" is similar for the cultural groups studied, it is important to note that factor analysis can only confirm those domains that have been put forth for confirmation. An instrument developed in one country could easily miss important domains in another; this would not be revealed in factor analysis.

Criterion validity refers to the correspondence between a proposed measure and another measure of the same variable taken to be a more accurate, or criterion variable. Criterion validity is the most prized type of validity. No "gold standard" exists, however, for most behavioral and perception-based quality of life measures. Some investigators suggest adopting an existing measure as the gold standard against which to compare other measures. There is no basis, however, for identifying a single measure that can serve as such a criterion. In this field, like most areas of social science, construct validation is necessary.

Construct validity is a term used to connote the use of theory in guiding the comparison of measures or groups to assess the validity of a measure. The major method used to provide evidence of construct validity is to compare one measure to another. This involves specifying the factors, or constructs, that account for variance in the proposed measures as well as the hypothesized relations among them. Hypotheses are stated regarding the direction and, if possible, the strength of relationships that might be expected. Validity is supported when the associations are consistent with prior hypotheses.

The construct validity of some generic health status measures has been established, although no general theory of expected differences has emerged (Patrick and Erickson 1993). The construct validity of disease-specific measures is less well established and cross-cultural use of construct validation is in its infancy.

Discriminant and convergent validity are types of construct validity. If different measures of the same construct are logically related and highly correlated, then convergent validity has been achieved. If a logically different measure is not as highly correlated as a more related measure, then discriminant validity is evident. Campbell and Fiske (1959) proposed the multitrait-multimethod procedure for evaluating the convergent and discriminant validity of measures.

Different measures of the same trait should show a strong, positive correlation (convergent) and weaker correlations with different traits (discriminant).

Convergent validity for the herpes-specific instrument will be assessed using a self-regard subscale from Fleming's Self-esteem scale (Fleming and Courtney 1984). It is hypothesized that the total quality of life score on the herpes-specific instrument will correlate positively with the self-regard score from the Fleming Self-esteem scale. Convergent validity has proven to be problematic even within the U.S. because of the lack of an established "stigma" scale. Based on the literature review and ethnographic interviews, "stigma" may have been a better concept to use than self-esteem. Moreover, cross-cultural attempts at assessing construct validity are usually impossible because of the lack of parallel instruments available in all cultures. Consequently, convergent and discriminant validity are often tested uniquely in each country.

Known groups validity is a type of discriminant validity that involves demonstrating that a measure can differentiate members of one group from another (DeVellis 1991). Known groups validity has been used in bivariate analyses with other quality of life data, such as the Medical Outcomes Study – Short Form-36 (MOS SF-36) (Sherbourne and Meredith 1992). The purpose may be either theory-related or to predict scores for one measure from another, usually a shorter instrument. In the first case, the procedure is a form of construct validity and, in the latter, criterion-related validity (DeVellis 1991). Linear regression and analysis of variance methods are useful in assessing known-groups validity.

In assessing the validity of the herpes measure, biological similarities of the condition across cultures were taken into account. After consulting with clinicians and researchers specializing in genital herpes, there was consensus that quality of life would be associated with clinical status. More specifically, the quality of life score on the herpes-specific measure should be inversely correlated with the frequency and severity of outbreaks. Analysis of covariance will be used to test this hypothesis. Using a retrospective cohort design, participants are being recruited based on the number of outbreaks experienced in the past year.

Three groups have been chosen for comparison of quality of life scores based on the number of outbreaks in the past year: 1) those with no outbreaks; 2) those with one to three; and 3) those with four or more. After controlling for potential confounders, such as age and gender, the "number of outbreaks" will be entered into a regression model as a dummy variable; the same will be done for "severity of outbreaks". A multiplicative interaction term will be tested as well. Solving the regression equation for the dependent variable (QOL score) will produce a mean QOL score for each subgroup. Results of the partial F-test for the number of outbreaks will be interpreted as support or lack of support for discriminant validity.

Discriminant validity has intuitive appeal in that data collection on the number and severity of outbreaks, and their hypothesized association with quality of life, seems straightforward, even at a cross-cultural level. Discriminant validity also addresses a key issue in clinical trials: might a therapy that reduced or altogether suppressed outbreaks of genital herpes affect quality of life? A statistical model that incorporates laboratory or clinical independent variables also may lend credibility to an instrument among clinicians.

One caveat is that biology is not always as similar as it might seem. For example, people in European and African countries are less likely to experience the same severity of symptoms as Americans because of differences in Herpes Simplex Virus Type I seroprevalence (Nahmias 1990). The wider (almost universal) exposure to HSV-1 outside of the United States prevents many cases of Herpes Simplex Virus Type II from ever becoming symptomatic, or if symptomatic, at least less severe. This variation may not be problematic as long as culture is controlled for in analyses combining data from several cultures.

Responsiveness

The ability of an instrument to detect small but important changes can be referred to as its responsiveness (Guyatt et al. 1987), although some investigators prefer to consider this a type of validity for assessing change. Advance knowledge of a measure's responsiveness aids in selecting measures, permits accurate estimation of sample size to assure sufficient statistical power, and assists in prioritizing or reducing the number of endpoints to be assessed.

Population or condition-specific measures can be more responsive than generic measures, because they tap domains of particular interest to persons with the condition, whereby small changes may be more easily detected. For a measure to detect subtle but important changes, scores must be stable among persons who are stable (reproducible), and changing among persons who experience actual change, however slight that change may be.

Different methods are available for measuring the responsiveness of a measure. Perhaps the most common method is to compare instrument scores before and after treatment of known efficacy. An improvement in scores would be evidence of responsiveness, as evaluated using the paired t-test statistic for within-subject changes. A second method for comparing responsiveness is to calculate "effect size" – the changes in mean score from base line to follow up divided by the standard deviation of base line scores (Kazis et al. 1989), or the standard deviation of score changes among stable subjects (Guyatt et al. 1987). The third method is based on the Receiver Operating Characteristic (ROC) curve most often applied to diagnostic technologies. Changes on a health status instrument are viewed as diagnostic tests for patient improvement, and the investigator seeks to distinguish between those who improve and those who do not (Deyo et al. 1991).

Because of increasing use of quality of life measures in longitudinal investigations, researchers are giving more attention to responsiveness. When responsiveness is important but suboptimal, several methods are available for improving it. Some proposals include using finer response categories, disaggregating scores, using specific transition questions ("much better" to "much worse"), and showing respondents their previous responses (Guyatt et al. 1989). For the herpes-specific instrument a sample of individuals will complete the instrument while in an outbreak, and again three weeks later when the outbreak is over. This offers an assessment of the acute impact of genital herpes on a person's quality of life.

Effect Size Interpretation

A measurement issue related to responsiveness is the calculation and interpretation of change scores in quality of life measures. Effect size is an estimate of change in health-related quality of life. Effect sizes translate the before-and-after changes into a standardized statistic to account for within-subject and between-subject variation. Effect sizes must be interpreted, and this can be accomplished using global ratings of change and the perceived importance of these changes, relating effects to treatments of known effectiveness, relating changes to clinical measures or clinical condition, or interpreting observed changes in terms of elements of those measures more meaningful to clinicians, policy-makers, and others using measures. Effect sizes for generic measures are usually established over a long period of using the measure resulting in a consensus on what constitutes a significant change score or effect size, e.g., a 3-point or 5-point change in the Sickness Impact Profile (Patrick and Erickson 1993). In contrast, the meaning of effect size for condition-specific instruments must be determined as part of its development process, often with limited data. Because the quality of life measures are usually analyzed as continuous variables, it is not hard to achieve "statistical significance" even in modest samples. For this reason, it is important that a change defined by the effect statistic have interpretational, clinical, or policy relevance.

One method for assessing the clinical meaningfulness of an effect is to compare changes seen in a quality of life measure to other clinical changes or results (Lydick and Epstein 1993). For example, a quality of life change associated with treatment of epilepsy might be interpreted in relation to the frequency or cessation of seizure. Another commonly reported "anchor-based" interpretation suggested by Jaeschke et al. (1989) is based on a patient and/or clinician global rating question. In this case, the changes seen in a disease-specific questionnaire are "anchored" to reported changes in overall health status. The clinically meaningful differences can be expressed in changes in the total questionnaire score or changes per item.

An interesting approach reported by Testa et al. (1993) is to correlate observed life events seen in a population of hypertensive men with changes in a concomitantly administered quality of life battery. In this study, the quality of life instruments detected changes that corresponded to moderately stressful life events. This method assumes that major life events are easier to understand than changes in the quality of life measure and that changes associated with hypertensive treatment can be associated with stress as a result of the life event, i.e., losing a job, getting a divorce, or having a child.

For the herpes specific measure, the effect size will be calculated as the difference in the quality of life score between the onset of an outbreak of herpes and the relief of symptoms at a later date, approximately three weeks from the onset of the outbreak. This interpretation will have clear meaning to patients and clinicians, although it may not be easily interpreted by persons who have never experienced herpes. Persons experiencing relief from a herpes outbreak will also be asked to rate their change in quality of life on a 7-point scale ranging from "much better" to "much worse." Changes in the herpes-specific measure will then be calibrated to these global ratings.

Cross-cultural interpretation of effect sizes will depend on the comparability of standards for interpretation. Life events, for example, may not have similar cultural meaning and could prove difficult to use in interpreting effect sizes observed in different countries. Global ratings of change could be influenced by cultural differences in the "anchoring" of changes, in that cultures may not discriminate small, medium, and large changes in the same way. Relating changes in the quality of life measure to changes in clinical status and using global ratings of change from the patients themselves are most likely to achieve cross-cultural comparability in understanding of effect sizes.

Conclusions

Cross-cultural validation of quality of life measures is an ongoing process of repeated application of theory and measurement. The most desirable means of validation is to approach instrument development with the goal of cross-cultural comparability in mind. Measures developed simultaneously in different cultures have the advantage of identifying as early as possible those domains and items that are more or less valid in a particular culture or population. Translating instruments developed in one culture for use in another is more common, most often because of the time and resources necessary to develop measures simultaneously in different cultures. The dangers of translation, however, are that the conceptual structure and domains contained in the instrument may not be sufficiently comprehensive for all cultures in which the measure is to be used.

Once translated or developed simultaneously, the next challenge is to test the reproducibility, validity, and responsiveness of the instrument in each culture. It is important that the methodology for assessment be standardized across cultures as much as possible. In addition to these methodological barriers, practical challenges include commitment of sufficient resources and frequent communication among investigators. Recruitment of comparable samples of persons on which to test quality of life measures in each country is also a major challenge.

Overcoming the conceptual, methodological, and practical barriers to cross-cultural validation will require a higher level of cooperation and coordination of investigative sites in the different countries participating in instrument development. To achieve conceptual and semantic equivalence and to improve standardization of validation procedures require agreement on field test protocols, adherence to these protocols, and frequent communication among sites on problems and solutions. A wider range of populations representing different subgroups of national populations need to be included in validation studies. Such studies are expensive, and development of cross-culturally valid instruments requires considerable investment on the part of study sponsors. Such investment will be necessary to achieve the standardization of measurement procedures and comparability and interpretation of outcomes.

As the development of cross-cultural measures of quality of life becomes more specialized, expertise on assuring reliability, validity, and responsiveness of these measures will improve. The use of these measures will aid in the quest for information that is relevant and informative to cultures around the world.

Acknowledgments

This work has been sponsored in part by grants from the Upjohn Company, Burroughs Wellcome, Inc. and the Wellcome Foundation.

References

Aday LA (1989) Designing and Conducting Health Surveys. Jossey-Bass Publishers, San Francisco

Bardo JW, Hughey JB (1984) The structure of community satisfaction in a British and an American community. J Social Psychol 124(2):151–157

Campbell DT, Fiske DW (1959) Convergent and discriminant validation by the multitrait–multimethod matrix. Psychol Bull 56:85–105

Corey L (1989) Genital herpes. In: Holmes K (ed). Sexually transmitted diseases. New York, McGraw-Hill Information Services Company

Del Greco L, Walop W, Eastridge L (1987) Questionnaire Development 3. Translation. Can Med Assoc 136:817–818

DeVellis RF (1991) Scale Development: Theory and Application. Applied Social Research Methods Series, Vol 26. Newbury Park, London, New Delhi, Sage Publications.

Deyo RA, Diehr P, Patrick DL (1991) Reproducibility and responsiveness of health status measures: statistics and strategies for evaluation. Controlled Clin Trials. 12:142S–158S

Fabrega H (1974) Disease and social behavior: an interdisciplinary perspective. Cambridge, Massachusetts Institute of Technology Press

Fleming JS, Courtney BE (1984) The dimensionality of self-esteem: II. Hierarchial facet model for revised measurement scales. J Personality Social Psych 46(2):404–421

Guinot P, Wesnes K (1985) A quality of life scale for the elderly: validation by factor analysis. IRCS Med Sci Psychol Psychiat 13:9–10

Guyatt G, Walter S, Norman G (1987) Measuring change over time: assessing the usefulness of evaluative instruments. J Chronic Dis 40(2):171–178

Guyatt GH, Deyo RA, Charlson M, Levine MN, Mitchell A (1989) Responsiveness and validity in health status measurement: a clarification. J Clin Epidemiol 42(5):403–408

Hunt SM (1993) Cross-cultural comparability of quality of life measures. Drug Info J 1993; 27:395–400

Hunt SM, McKenna S (1992) The QLDS: A scale for the measurement of quality of life in depression. Health Policy 22:307–319

Jaeschke R, Singer J, Guyatt GH (1989) Measurement of health status: ascertaining the minimal clinically important difference. Control Clin Trial 10:407–415

Jobe JB, Mingay DJ (1989) Cognitive research improves questionnaires. Am J Public Health. 79(8):1053–1055

Kazis LE, Anderson JJ, Meenan RF (1989) Effect sizes for interpreting changes in health status. Med Care 27 (3 suppl):S178–S189

Kleinman A, Eisenberg L, Good B (1978) Culture, illness and care: clinical lessons from anthropologic and cross-cultural research. Ann Int Med 88:251–258

Lydick E, Epstein RS (1993) Interpretation of quality of life changes. Quality Life Res 2(3):221–226

Nahmias AJ, Lee FK, Beckman-Nahmias S (1990) Sero-epidemiological and sociological patterns of herpes simplex virus infection in the world. Scand J Infect Dis Suppl 69:19–36

Nunnally JC (1978) Psychometric theory, 2nd ed. New York, McGraw-Hill

Patrick DL, Erickson P (1993) Health status and health policy: allocating resources to health care. New York, Oxford University Press

Sartorius N (1993) A WHO method for the assessment of health-related quality of life (WHOQOL). In: Walker SR and Rosser RM (eds). Quality of life assessment: key issues in the 1990's. Boston, Kluwer Academic Publishers, pp 201–207

Sherbourne CD, Meredith LS (1992) Quality of self-report data: a comparison of older and younger chronically ill patients. J Gerontol Social Sci 47(4):S204–S211

Stewart AL, Ware JE (eds) (1992) Measuring functioning and well-being. The Medical Outcomes Study Approach. Durham and London, Duke University Press

Testa MA, Anderson RB, Nackley JF, Hollenberg NK (1993) Quality of life and antihypertensive therapy in men: a comparison of Captopril with Enalapril. New Engl J Med 328(13):907–913

Ware JE (1987) Standards for validating health measures: definition and content. J Chronic Dis 40(6):473–480

Wellcome Dialog (1992) Informational Booklet on Genital Herpes. Burroughs Welcome Co

WHOQOL Group (1993) Study protocol for the World Health Organization project to develop a Quality of Life Instrument (WHOQOL). Quality Life Res 2:153–159

Ensuring International Equivalence of Quality of Life Measures: Problems and Approaches to Solutions

M. Bullinger

Summary

Equivalence of international versions of a quality of life measure is vital to its use in research. Along the lines of an approach proposed in cross-cultural psychology, the functional, scale, operational and metric equivalence criteria are outlined and elaborated using translation and testing of the SF-36 as an example. The problems faced in examining and meeting these criteria, as well as possible procedural solutions, are discussed.

Introduction

Problems of international validation of health status measures are similar to those encountered in any scientific attempt to work cross-culturally with a standard measurement system. Contrary to the majority of outcome assessments in the life sciences, the relative cross-cultural stability or invariance of a measurement system in the social and behavioral sciences cannot be assumed. This is because relevant endpoints in this area often pertain to the attitudinal orientations, cognitive evaluations or emotional states of the respondents, which are assumed to be culturally diverse (Dressler et al. 1991; Kleinman et al. 1978).

Basically, such phenomena are constructs that need to be defined and operationalized in a conceptual model before an attempt is made to measure them. Quality of life can be viewed as referring to well-being and functioning in the physical, emotional, mental, social and everyday life domains as experienced by the respondent (Bullinger 1991). These domains can be addressed by obtaining relevant information via interviews or questionnaires.

While there is international agreement on the prerequisites for quality of life assessment in terms of concepts and methods, this agreement only pertains to quality standards of instruments within cultures, not necessarily across cultures. In each culture, especially the Anglo-American, various instruments for quality of life assessment have been proposed that fulfill the above-mentioned quality criteria (McDowell and Newell 1987). In the age of increased international collaboration in medical research, however, a strong interest has developed in quality of life instruments available in different multi-national

J. Orley, W. Kuyken (Eds.)
Quality of Life Assessment:
International Perspectives

research projects (Walker and Rosser 1992). Necessary steps to ensure the international applicability of instruments already available in one language include the translation and psychometric testing of instruments (Bullinger and Hasford 1991).

Interestingly, in spite of increasing literature on the use of quality of life questionnaires in different countries and in spite of the growing cross-cultural research area, very few papers deal directly with methodological criteria for developing and evaluating quality of life measures internationally (Hunt 1993; Sartorius 1987; Bullinger et al. 1993). A fruitful approach, even though not specific to quality of life measures, was proposed by Hui and Triandis (1985), who postulated four dimensions of equivalence when attempting to measure a construct (such as quality of life) internationally. These dimensions are:

1) functional equivalence – whether the items in the translated language version of a scale have a meaning similar to that in the source version;
2) scale equivalence – the extent to which individuals in different cultural groups respond to similar items in similar ways;
3) operational equivalence – the comparability of procedures used in obtaining the needed information, including comparisons of psychometric instrument performance; and
4) scalar or metric equivalence – whether a measure orders individuals along a continuum in a comparable way across language groups.

Most recently, an international quality of life working group (IQOLA) established a set of procedures for the translation and psychometric testing of the SF-36 (Aaronson et al. 1992). The SF-36 is the 36-item short form of the measures used in the Medical Outcome Study (Tarlov et al. 1989; Stewart and Ware 1992). It contains eight health concepts – namely physical functioning, role-physical functioning, role-emotional functioning, mental health, vitality, social functioning, pain and general health perception – and was intensively tested for psychometric performance in the USA. Because of its brevity and methodological quality it is currently regarded as one of the more promising generic, patient-based health outcome measures and has received increased attention (Ware 1993). Along the lines of the Hui and Triandis approach (1985), the problems encountered in the international work with the SF-36 involve the adequacy of translations, comparability of response scales, standardization of psychometric testing procedures and transferability of scoring results from one culture to another.

Functional Equivalence

The majority of problems encountered in this area involve a critical assessment of the translation. The question here is how well the translations (of instructions, items, responses) are performed, i.e., to establish a set of examination criteria. Although adherence to a predefined translation protocol is usually demanded, the question of how well the translation process was done tends to be left to informal group discussions and decisions or to post hoc empirical testing of the instrument's performance. Usually quality assessments of translations are not routinely done in a standard or quantifiable way.

For the SF-36, a forward-backward translation with quality ratings was developed (Aaronson et al. 1992; Bullinger et al. in preparation). This process includes two forward translations of the original instrument into the new language, where the two independent translators meet to agree on a common version which is then retranslated into English by two other translators, who also meet to agree on their retranslated version. Those agreed upon versions are then quality-rated for instructions, items and responses on a 0–100 (optimum) visual analogue scale according to "conceptual equivalence," "colloquial language use" and "parsimony" of the translations by a set of reviewers, so that the quality of the translation is explicitly assessed. Finally, the English retranslation is compared to the original by one of the persons who originally developed the instrument.

Use of this method in Germany, for example, resulted in a high quality of ratings (over 90 with high interrater agreement) on the vast majority of items, and responses with lower ratings (below 75) flagged translation problems (Bullinger 1994). The aim of this procedure, especially the formalized quantitative assessment by raters, is to have documented and analyzable information about the translation process which can be used as feedback on translation problems. According to this iterative procedure, low ratings on the three aforementioned dimensions would suggest going back to an earlier stage in the translation process and beginning anew. The care with which the translation process is performed and documented feeds directly into the next problem area, scale equivalence.

Scale Equivalence

An important step in the statistical validation of instruments is to ensure the cross-cultural comparability of response scales. An example of how to deal with this is given by the IQOLA project, in which the examination of the response choice in terms of a Thurstone scaling exercise was explicitly included.

To assess whether the response choices were ordinal and represented equidistantly within and across countries, each response choice was to be rated on a visual-analogue scale (VAS) ranging from the item representing the lowest scale limit (0 mm) to the item representing the highest scale limit (100 mm). All response choices were assembled with a VAS on one page in random order.

The ratings were done by a group of 50 persons per country, who positioned each response on the VAS line between the upper and lower scale limit; subsequently the average of that value per response across the group was calculated. The resulting 0–100 scores per item were then transformed to reflect the original order of responses (e.g. 1, 2, 3, 4, 5, on a 5-point Likert scale).

Assembling this information across countries provides possibilities of examining 1) the ordinality of responses, in that the country means should reflect the rank order of the original as well as the number of violations of that order per country; 2) the equidistance of responses, in that the country means should be close to the original numbers as well as the deviation from this original per country; and 3) the quality of response scale translations, in that violations of order and equidistance might reflect having chosen an inappropriate term for a specific response.

For Germany, ranks corresponded to the original sequence of responses, and distances between responses were similar to the US values. Having undertaken the Thurstone exercise in 10 IQOLA countries including the country of origin, USA, the results showed that, for the SF-36 responses, ordinality can be inferred in every country, whereas MANOVA results showed significant country differences in some of the distance assessments. This finding led to a revision of response scales in specific countries and to a discussion of recalibrating one of the original US scales (Bullinger et al., in preparation).

Operational Equivalence

Operational equivalence pertains to 1) the standardization of the testing procedures employed in each country and the identification of respondent groups in which to do the testing, as well as technical standardization of the process via a study protocol and 2) an a priori definition of criteria, statistical procedures and decisions about the instrument quality across nations.

Psychometric performance criteria for psychological measures in general and specifically for quality of life instruments have been described repeatedly. They involve classical psychometric criteria such as reliability and validity (Nunally 1978; Ware 1987) but, for the evaluative purpose of quality of life assessment, the additional criterion of responsiveness to change or sensitivity is of special importance (Guyatt et al. 1989; Patrick et al., this volume).

Critical values include good variance of items, item/scale validity in terms of optimal scale fit, item to scale correlations above $r = 0.40$, internal consistency coefficients over alpha = 0.70, correlations coefficients for convergent validity testing of above $r = 0.50$, discriminant validity in terms of distinguishing between clinically different groups, clear factor structures replicating the original scales with the same items and the explanation of comparable variances.

A set of problems concerns the specific cut-off points according to which an instrument is reliable or unreliable. Usually for internal consistency, for example, the Cronbach Alpha coefficient of over alpha = 0.70 is considered necessary to confirm reliability of the scale. However, in some research contexts lower reliability might be acceptable because the scale meets other performance criteria, such as precision or differentiating between specific groups. Thus, the psychometric criteria should not be used in a textbook fashion but should be adapted to the purpose of the instrument in a given national or international study (Bullinger and Hasford, 1991).

International examination of psychometric performance is more complicated. The question here is which set of criteria should be employed to infer the international validity and reliability of an instrument. One approach towards establishing international psychometric quality would be to simply assemble for each country all available information on reliability, validity and sensitivity of an instrument and use the classical cut-off points for instrument performance obtained from each nation. One could argue that, if in a given country under diverse conditions an instrument continues to show excellent psychometric properties, it can be assumed to be culturally acceptable. Thus, by assembling information from different nations, international comparability could be inferred. This sounds easy and certainly is often adopted.

However, a pitfall may be a comparison between "apples and pears," because studies often have not been designed to be internationally comparable with regard to patient population, study design and intervention. A minimum requirement, therefore, should be to have at least one or two patient groups in study designs between different countries that are so comparable that psychometric performance criteria can be tied to specific populations and trial designs across cultures.

The most elegant but also most complicated approach would be the a priori design of an international validation study which assures that the patient population studies designs employed and the measures taken are equivalent. The EORTC Quality of Life working group has adopted this approach in testing the EORTC QLQ in different countries according to a predefined study protocol (Aaronson et al. 1991). Such a study design ideally mimics the design of a multi-national clinical trial, including a well-written study protocol with a clear procedural section and a comprehensive statistical analysis part. Such an approach is only realizable, however, in an international research setting with substantial support in terms of government-funded cross-national epidemiological trials or industry-sponsored multi-national trials of a specific compound.

Scalar or Metric Equivalence

This step can only be reached after the preceding three have been successfully completed. For example, placing two tested individuals from different countries with an identical score on a scale assumes that this scale (e.g., mental health subscale score) reflects the same degree of impairment in both countries. Before making this assumption it is necessary to ascertain that the two scores in fact represent the identical degree of impairment. This can be tested by obtaining ratings of the health states included in the questionnaire by health experts, an approach followed, for example, in the work with the Nottingham Health Profile (Hunt and Wiklund 1987). A second option is to include the questionnaire in a representative study yielding norms of the measure, which is carried out after the instrument development and aims to obtain reference data from a representative population sample. Thus, norms from different countries can be used to determine scale scores internationally. Such a weighing approach is increasingly employed in health economic research on quality of life (Patrick and Erickson 1993). As an extension, weighing judgements could also be made by a representative sample of the population, i.e., by including the weighing procedure in the norming process.

An alternative way, similar to convergent validation, is to test whether scores of two individuals would also be similar on another measure of mental health or if changes over time were comparable. This of course assumes that scores on the two measures have a linear relationship. The scalar equivalence is strictly necessary in clinical trials or epidemiological studies in which data are pooled across countries. A lenient approach would not insist on demonstration of scalar equivalence if analyses were carried out country by country. Thus the decision about scalar equivalence depends on the nature of the trials planned with an instrument.

In general, the more sophisticated the criteria to be fulfilled by an instrument are, the more comprehensive and standardized the research on the instrument has to be when planned, carried out and examined.

Conclusion

The process of developing and evaluating quality of life measures is an iterative one. The question arises as to what extent the evaluation and psychometric testing in a national context might lead to a change in the original concept, the original instrument or the methodological approach chosen for instrument development. While this is still an open question, and is associated with the risk of loosing large data-sets for reference in comparison with actual results, allowing such modification might be a wise decision. Incongruencies in translations or psychometric problems with scales detected in single nations might lead to a further refinement of the instrument for use in international research or to the acknowledgement of nation-specific versions of instruments.

In general the line between a correctly translated version or an adapted version of an original instrument is not easily drawn. Slight modifications in the wording or choice of examples (e.g., "moderate activities" in the functional limitation scale of the SF-36: picking berries in Sweden versus playing golf in America) might be considered as allowed colloquial variations on the theme rather than forbidden changes of the original item. Basically, one way to critically assess the impact of such slight modifications is the inspection of statistical characteristics, such as item distributions and reliability coefficients. Should, for example, the percentage of the Americans agreeing to playing golf differ from Swedish berry picking, a problem in item comparability would be detected. Thus translation and evaluation are really interdependent steps in the process of generating an internationally valuable scale.

Even though those precautions do not speak against attempting to develop and internationally evaluate quality of life measures, they do imply that the development and evaluation process has to be clear-cut, well-planned, organized and standardized in procedures, with statistical analysis defined a priori (Bullinger et al., in preparation). Minimal requirements for inferring correct translation and international evaluation of an instrument are the forward-backward translation in each language under study, a test of psychometric criteria for both healthy and ill persons in a country, including at least 100 patients per study, and a clear-cut description of that translation and evaluation process. The optimal requirement would be to include a more refined translation process using more translators, focus groups and response scaling for evaluation. An optimum for testing would involve having on hand a well-designed and formulated study protocol to conduct a cross-cultural evaluation of an instrument (very much like a multi-national clinical trial protocol) and the use of innovative statistical procedures to compare the quality of test criteria obtained and international comparability (e.g., testing the significance of differences between the psychometric indicators within the same population across cultures).

Although the optimum requires conceptual work as well as practical possibilities to conduct such research, it should serve as a goal and lead researchers to move from fulfillment of the more basic requirements to more sophisticated approaches to develop and evaluate quality of life measures internationally.

Acknowledgements

The work of the IQOLA group regarding the international translation and testing of the SF-36 health outcome measure was taken as an example in this paper. Members of the IQOLA group are N. Aaronson, C. Acquadro, I. Alonso, G. Apolone, D. Bucquet, M. Bullinger, K. Bungay, S. Fukuhara, B. Gandek, S. Keller, A. Leplege, D. Razavi, R. Sanson-Fisher, M. Sullivan, S. Wood-Dauphinee, A. Wagner and J. Ware Jr.

References

Aaronson N, Ahmedzai S, Bullinger M, Crabeels D, Estapè J, Filiberti A, Flechtner H, Frick U, Hürny C, Kaasa S, Klee M, Mastilicia M, Osoba D, Pfausler B, Razavi D, Rofe P, Schraub S, Sullivan M, Takeda F (1991) The EORTC Core quality of life questionnaire: interim results of an international field study. In: Osoba D (ed) Effect of cancer on quality of life. CRC Press, Vancouver, pp 136–154

Aaronson, N, Acquadro C, Alonso J, Apolone G, Bucquet D, Bullinger M, Bungay K, Fukuhara S, Gandek B, Keller S, Razavi D, Sanson-Fisher R, Sullivan M, Wood-Dauphinee S, Wagner A, Ware J (1992) International quality of life assessment (IQOLA) project. Quality Life Res 1:349–351

Bullinger M (1991) Quality of life – definition, conceptualization and implications – a methodologist's view. Theoretical Surg 6:143–148

Bullinger M (1994) German translation and psychometric testing of the SF-36 – preliminary results from the IQOLA Project. Social Sci Med, in press

Bullinger M, Hasford J (1991) Evaluating quality of life measures. German clinical trials. Controlled Clin Trials 12:915–1055

Bullinger M, Cella D, Aaronson N, Anderson R (1993) Developing and evaluating cross-national instruments from minimum requirements to optimal models. Quality Life Res 2:451–459

Dressler WW, Vieteri, FE, Chavez A, Greel GAC, Dos Santos JE (1991) Comparative research in social epidemiology: measurement issues. Ethnicity Disease 1:379–393

Guyatt GH, Deyo RA, Charlson M, Levine MN, Mitchell A (1989) Responsiveness and validity in health status measurement: a clarification. J Clin Epidemiol 42(5):403–408

Hui CH, Triandis HC (1985) Measurement in cross-cultural psychology: a review and comparison of strategies. J Cross-Cultural Psychol 16(2):131–152

Hunt SM (1993) Cross-cultural comparability of quality of life measures. Drug Info J 27:395–400

Hunt SM, Wiklund I (1987) Cross-cultural variation in the weighting of health statements: a comparison of English and Swedish valuations. Health Pol 8:227–235

Kleinman A, Eisenberg L, Good B (1978) Culture, illness and care: clinical lessons from anthropologic and cross-cultural research. Ann Int Med 88:251–258

McDowell I, Newell C (1987) Measuring health: A guide to rating scales and questionnaires. Oxford University Press, New York

Nunnally JC (1978) Psychometric theory. 2nd ed. New York, Mc Graw-Hill

Patrick DL, Erikson P (1993) Health status and health policy: Allocating resources to health care. Oxford University Press, New York

Sartorius N (1987) Cross cultural comparisons of data about quality of life: a sample of issues. In: Aaronson NK, Beckmann J (eds) The quality of life of cancer patients. Raven Press, New York, pp 1075–1077

Stewart AL, Ware JE (eds) (1992) Measuring functioning ans well-being: the Medical Outcomes Study approach. Duke University Press, Durham and London

Tarlov A, Ware J, Greenfield S, Nelson E, Perrin E, Zubkoff M (1989) The Medical Outcome Study: an application of methods for monitoring the results of medical care. JAMA 262:925–930

Walker S, Rosser R (1992) Quality of life: key issues in the 1990s. Kluwer Academic Press, Dordrecht

Ware JE (1987) Standards for validating health measures: definition and content. J Chronic Dis 40(6):473–480

Ware JE (1993) The SF-36 Health Survey – Manual and interpretation guide. New England Medical Center (Health Institute). Nimrod Press, Boston

The Development of the World Health Organization Quality of Life Assessment Instrument (the WHOQOL)

The WHOQOL Group[1]

The World Health Organization (WHO) is developing an international quality of life assessment instrument (WHOQOL) which will allow an enquiry into the perception of individuals of their own position in life in the context of the culture and value systems in which they live, and in relation to their goals, expectations, standards and concerns. The WHOQOL will measure quality of life related to health and health care. It is being developed in the framework of a collaborative project involving numerous centres in different cultural settings. In addition it will have proven psychometric properties of validity, reliability and responsiveness to change and will be sensitive to the cultural setting in

[1] This paper was drafted by Dr. Willem Kuyken and Dr. John Orley on behalf of the WHOQOL Group. The WHOQOL group comprises a coordinating group, collaborating investigators in each of the field centres, and a panel of consultants. Responsible staff at headquaters in WHO, Geneva, are: Dr. J. Orley, Dr. W. Kuyken and Dr. N. Sartorius. In the field centres collaborating investigators are: Professor H. Herrman, Dr. H. Schofield and Ms. B. Murphy, University of Melbourne, Australia; Professor Z. Metelko, Professor S. Szabo and Mrs. Pibernik-Okanovic, Institute of Diabetes, Endocrinology and Metabolic Diseases and Department of Psychology, Faculty of Philosophy, University of Zagreb, Croatia; Dr. N. Quemada and Dr. A. Caria, INSERM, Paris, France; Dr. S. Rajkumar and Mrs. Shuba Kumar, Madras Medical College, India; Dr. S. Saxena, All India Institute of Medical Sciences, Delhi, India; Dr. D. Bar-On and Dr. M. Amir, Ben-Gurion University, Beer-Sheeva, Israel; Dr. Professor Dr. G. Van Heck and Mrs. J. De Vries, Tilburg University, The Netherlands; Professor J. Arroyo Sucre, University of Panama, Panama; Professor M. Kabanov, Dr. A. Lomachenkov and Dr. G. Burkovsky, Bekhterev Psychoneurological Research Institute, St. Petersburg, Russia; Professor Sompotch Sukwatana and Mr. Kitikorn Meesapya, Institute of Mental Health, Bangkok, Thailand; Dr. S. Skevington, Ms. P. MacArthur and Ms. M. Somerset, University of Bath, United Kingdom; Dr. D. Patrick, Ms. M. Martin and Ms. D. Wild, University of Washington, Seattle, USA and Professor W. Acuda, Dr. J. Mutambirwa, University of Zimbabwe, Harare, Zimbabwe. Further centres in China, Japan and Spain are likely to join the project in the coming months. The project is sponsored by WHO and is funded by WHO, the participating field centres, the Carnegie Foundation, the IPSEN Foundation, and the Upjohn Company.

The consultants that have advised WHO at various stages of the development of the project have included: Dr. N.K. Aaronson, Dr. P. Bech, Dr. N. Blinov, Dr. D. Bueshing, Dr. D. Bucquet, Dr. M. Bullinger, Dr. L.W. Chambers, Dr. He-Nian Chen, Dr. B. Cramer, Dr. B. Jambon, Dr. C.D. Jenkins, Dr. D. De Leo, Dr. L. Fallowfield, Dr. J. Fox-Rushby, Dr. P. Gerin, Dr. P. Graham, Dr. O. Gureje, Dr. R. Hays, Dr. K. Kalumba, Dr. Kerr-Correa, Dr. L. Kogan, Dr. C. Mercier, Dr. C. Moinpour, Mr. J. Oliver, Dr. Y.H. Poortinga, Dr. R. Rosser, Dr. R. Trotter and Dr. F. Van Dam.

Further information can be obtained from the WHOQOL Group, Division of Mental Health, World Health Organization, CH-1211 Geneva 27, Switzerland.

which it is applied, while maintaining comparability of scores across different cultural settings. This chapter outlines the methodology for the development of the instrument and sets out the characteristics and uses of the WHOQOL.

WHO's initiative to develop a quality of life assessment arose for a number of reasons. In recent years there has been a broadening in focus in the measurement of health, beyond traditional health indicators such as mortality and morbidity (e.g., World Bank 1993; WHO 1991), to include measures of the impact of disease and impairment on daily activities and behaviour (e.g., Sickness Impact Profile; Bergner et al. 1981), perceived health measures (e.g., Nottingham Health Profile; Hunt et al. 1989) and disability/functional status measures (e.g., the MOS SF-36; Ware et al. 1993). These measures, whilst beginning to provide a measure of the impact of disease, do not assess quality of life *per se*, which has been aptly described as "the missing measurement in health" (Fallowfield 1990). Second, most measures of health status have been developed in North America and the UK, and the translation of these measures for use in other settings is time-consuming and unsatisfactory for a number of reasons (see Sartorius and Kuyken, this volume). Third, the increasingly mechanistic model of medicine, concerned *only* with the eradication of disease and symptoms, reinforces the need for the introduction of a humanistic element into health care. Health care is essentially a humanistic transaction in which the patient's well-being is a primary aim. By calling for quality of life assessments in health care, attention is focused on this aspect of health, and resulting interventions will pay increased attention to the problem. WHO's initiative to develop a quality of life assessment arises, therefore from a need for a genuinely international measure of quality of life and restates its commitment to the continued promotion of a holistic approach to health and health care.

The Development of the WHOQOL

This section outlines the principles and methods followed by WHO in its multi-centre collaborative project to develop an international quality of life assessment (WHO 1993c; WHOQOL Group 1993). This involved first establishing an approach to quality of life assessment (WHO 1992a, b), developing an agreed upon and detailed study protocol (WHO 1993b, c), and following a series of steps leading to a reliable, valid and responsive quality of life assessment. The steps involved operationalizing the domains and facets of quality of life, question and response scale generation, piloting work with a preliminary version of the instrument, development of the instrument on the basis of these data, and a series of reliability, validity and responsiveness studies.

A key feature of the methodology is the use of an iterative process of input from health professionals and quality of life researchers from around the world, cross-cultural lay review (through the use of focus groups), and international expert review. A unique feature of the project is that the WHOQOL instrument is being developed simultaneously in a wide range of languages and cultures. Field centres have been selected to provide differences in their levels of industrialization, available health services, and other markers relevant to the measurement of quality of life (e.g., role of the family, perception of time, perception of self, dominant religious denomination). Work on the development of the instrument has involved a central coordinating group (WHO Geneva), numerous field centres, and a panel of consultants who have advised the project throughout its development. The guidelines governing this collaboration are described elsewhere (Sartorius 1988).

Defining Quality of Life

The picture of health yielded by existing measures of health status (see McDowell and Newell 1987; Quality of Life Bibliography and Indexes 1990; Bowling 1991; Walker and Rosser 1993), often erroneously referred to as quality of life, is extremely useful but by no means complete. The individual's subjective evaluation of disease, impairment and disability is what can be termed "health-related quality of life." We suggest that health-related quality of life should broaden the focus of enquiry beyond symptomatology (e.g., location and nature of pain; presence and degree of fatigue) and effects of health/disease/illness on functional status (e.g., Can you walk several blocks/half a mile/a kilometre?), to include the person's subjective evaluation (e.g., How afraid are you of experiencing pain? How satisfied are you with the energy that you have? How happy are you with your ability to move around?).

We suggest, therefore, that the traditional conception of health-related quality of life misses the positive dimensions of well-being, as well as the complexity of what is meant by the terms "perceived,", "subjective," or "evaluative" (e.g., Gerin et al. 1992; Patrick and Erikson 1993).

Quality of life is defined, therefore, as an individual's perception of his/her position in life in the context of the culture and value systems in which he/she lives, and in relation to his/her goals, expectations, standards and concerns. It is a broad-ranging concept, incorporating in a complex way the person's physical health, psychological state, level of independence, social relationships, personal beliefs and relationship to salient features of the environment. This definition highlights the views that quality of life refers to a subjective evaluation, which induces both positive and negative dimensions, and which is embedded in a cultural, social and environmental context.

This definition of quality of life is consistent with WHO's definition of health as "a state of physical, mental and social well-being, not merely the absence of disease and infirmity." Because there is no standard scale for health, a broad range of health indicators is commonly used, each representing a domain of the overall concept. Similarly, in WHO's work on quality of life, six broad domains have been identified which describe core aspects of quality of life cross-culturally: a Physical domain (e.g., energy and fatigue), a Psychological domain (e.g., positive feelings), Level of independence, (e.g., mobility), Social relationships (e.g., practical social support), Environment (e.g., the accessibility of health care), and Personal beliefs/Spirituality (e.g., meaning in life). The domains of health and quality of life are clearly complementary and overlapping. For example, an assessment of patients' symptomatology (physical well-being) is complemented by an enquiry into the physical domain of quality of life, where questions address the patients' evaluation of their symptoms and their subjective reaction to any disability caused by the disease.

Operationalization of Domains and Facets of Quality of Life

Once an agreed-upon working definition of quality of life and study protocol were developed, a further phase of work involved operationalizing the broad domains and individual facets of quality of life for the WHOQOL instrument.

Consultants and principal investigators from each of the field centres drafted a provisional list of domains and constituent facets of quality of life (WHO 1992a, b). A definition for each facet of quality of life consisted of a conceptual definition, a description of various dimensions along which a rating can be made for that facet, and a listing of some example situations or conditions that might significantly affect that facet at various levels of intensity. Facets describe behaviours (e.g., activities as provider), states of being (e.g., fatigue), capacities (e.g., ability to move around) or subjective perceptions of experiences (e.g., pain).

Once facets of quality of life were drafted, a series of focus groups[2] were held with patients, well persons and health personnel in each of the field centres to consider the facet definitions drafted by health professionals and quality of life researchers. Each focus group comprised six to eight individuals, demographically representative of the target population in terms of gender, age, educational background, socioeconomic group and ethnic group. The procedure followed in the focus groups involved detailed orientation and instructions followed by a facet by facet discussion, in which participants were asked about how each facet affected their quality of life and how one might best ask about that facet. For the purposes of standardization, all primary focus group moderators were trained centrally at WHO, Geneva (WHO 1992c). The focus group data served to question the comprehensiveness and face validity of the facets of quality of life proposed for the WHOQOL. This process of facet operationalization ensures that the underlying dimensions of quality of life to

[2] Focus groups are essentially group interviews that are guided through skilful moderation towards a focused discussion on a topic. The comments and interactions between participants are transcribed and comprise the data. Focus groups are an important research tool for cross-cultural work. Their natural setting, their flexibility, and their semi-structured nature can yield rich data from widely different populations with standardised protocols (see Morgan 1988). Focus groups enabled a standardised methodology to be used to ask questions of "slum dwellers" in Madras, health personnel in Bangkok and patients in North America.

Table 1. WHOQOL facet definitions

Domain I – Physical domain	
1	Pain and discomfort
2	Energy and fatigue
3	Sexual activity
4	Sleep and rest
5	Sensory functions
Domain II – Psychological domain	
6	Positive feelings
7	Thinking, learning, memory and concentration
8	Self-esteem
9	Body image and appearance
10	Negative feelings
Domain III – Level of independence	
11	Mobility
12	Activities of daily living
13	Dependence on medicinal substances and medical aids
14	Dependence on non-medicinal substances (alcohol, tobacco, drug...)
15	Communication capacity
16	Work capacity
Domain IV – Social relationships	
17	Personal relationships
18	Practical social support
19	Activities as provider/supporter
Domain V – Environment	
20	Freedom, physical safety and security
21	Home environment
22	Work satisfaction
23	Financial resources
24	Health and social care: accessibility and quality
25	Opportunities for acquiring new information and skills
26	Participation in and opportunities for recreation/leisure activities
27	Physical environment (pollution/noise/traffic/climate)
28	Transport
Domain VI – Spirituality/Religion/Personal beliefs	

be enquired about are clearly defined, have high face validity, and have a core meaning that cuts across cultures.

On the basis of the focus group data, a revised set of facet definitions was compiled to guide subsequent item writing work (Table 1; WHO 1993a). As can be seen from Table 1, the WHOQOL provides a balanced and holistic assessment of a person's quality of life, where both positive and negative aspects of life are assessed together. The overall coverage of quality of life that results from this methodology ensures a conceptual coherence, or Gestalt, missing from many other measures of health status.

The definition of the facet *Self esteem* is given below, by way of illustrating the product of this process of facet operationalization.

Self esteem
This facet examines how the person feels about himself/herself as a person. This might range from feeling positive to feeling extremely negative about himself/herself. A person's sense of his/her worth as a person – whether he/she feels that he/she has any good qualities and his/her satisfaction with himself/herself – is explored. The aspect of self esteem concerned with a person's feeling of self-efficacy and control is also included in the focus of this facet.

Questions include the person's feelings about himself/herself in a range of areas: how he/she is able to get along with other people; his/her education; his/her appraisal of his/her ability to change or accomplish particular tasks or behaviours; family relations and the sense of dignity and self-acceptance that a person feels. To some people self-esteem depends largely on how they function, whether at work or at home, or how they are perceived and treated by others. In some cultures self-esteem is the esteem felt within the family rather than individual self-esteem.

Questions do not include very specific reference to body image, social relationships and work satisfaction as these are covered in different areas. However, the sense of self-worth that comes from these activities is intended to be covered by questions at a more general level.

It is acknowledged that some people may find self-esteem difficult to talk about, and questions are framed to take this into account.

Examples:
A person with clinical depression.
A person who is unable to find work.

Question Generation

After completion of the focus group work and after the WHOQOL facets of quality of life had been operationalized, a question-writing panel was assembled in each field centre. The question-writing panel included the principal investigator, the main focus group moderator, at least one person with good interviewing skills and experience, and a lay person, preferably someone who participated in one of the lay focus groups, to ensure that questions were framed in comprehensible and natural language.

Making full use of focus group transcripts the panel framed a maximum of six questions for each facet, at two levels of questioning; "perceived objective" (global evaluations of behaviour, states or capacities) and "self-report subjective" (perceived satisfaction/dissatisfaction with behaviours, states or capacities). Naturally questions were framed in the local language in which it was anticipated that the instrument would be used. Question-writing panels were instructed to use the criteria outlined in Table 2 in framing questions.

Through this process, the questions which comprise the WHOQOL can be said to originate with health personel and patients in each of the centres. This helps to ensure that questions are germane to the settings in which they will be asked, and that the questions for facets that are awkward, difficult to talk about, or taboo are suitable.

Questions from all centres were pooled to make up a "global question pool," comprising some 2000 questions. After duplicate questions had been identified and redundant questions removed, some 1800 questions remained. A content analysis of the questions, looking for semantically equivalent questions (e.g.,

Table 2. Criteria for WHOQOL questions

Questions should:

be based as far as possible on the suggestions of patients and health personnel participating in the focus groups;

give rise to answers that are illuminating about respondents' quality of life, as defined in the project;

be amenable to a rating scale;

reflect the meaning conveyed in the facet definition;

cover, in combination with other questions for a given facet, the key aspects of that facet as outlined in the facet definition;

avoid any explicit reference point in terms of time or in terms of comparison point(s) (e.g., the ideal, or before I was ill);

be applicable to patients with a range of impairments;

be phrased as questions rather than as statements;

be shorter rather than longer;

avoid double negatives; and,

avoid any ambiguities in terms of wording or phrasing.

"How much of the time are you tired?" and "How often are you tired?") which were subsequently treated as one question, reduced the number further. Questions were then carefully examined to see to what extent they met the criteria for WHOQOL questions (Table 2). This led to a considerable further reduction in the number of questions in the global pool to some 1000 questions. The principal investigator in each of the field centres then rank ordered the questions for each facet according to *"how much it tells you about a respondent's quality of life in your culture."* On the basis of the combined rankings from all centres 276 questions were selected for the WHOQOL pilot instrument.[3] The questions selected from this process for the *Self esteem* facet[4] were:

Perceived objective
1. How much do you value yourself?
2. How good do you feel about yourself?
3. How much confidence do you have in yourself?
4. Do you regard yourself as worthy of respect from others?

[3] The procedure for question selection is outlined in more detail in WHO, 1993c.

[4] Original language versions of these questions, or semantically equivalent versions, were generated in field centres in the following countries: question 1 – the Netherlands, Panama, UK, Zimbabwe; question 2 – Australia and USA; question 3 – France, the Netherlands and Thailand; question 4 – India; question 5 – Croatia and Panama; question 6 – Australia; question 7 – India.

Self-report subjective
5. How satisfied are you with yourself?
6. How satisfied are you with your abilities?
7. How satisfied are you with the respect you get from others?

Some facets of quality of life are relatively universal across cultures (e.g., *Mobility*), when compared to others such as *Self-esteem, Personal relationships* and *Spirituality/Religion/Personal beliefs.* Since the ranking by all centres may favour more global questions, some which address important, but culture-specific features of facets may have been omitted. Therefore, field centres were free to include two culture-specific questions per facet, which had been previously reviewed as meeting various quality control criteria (Table 2), to their national version of the pilot WHOQOL instrument. For example, in Thailand, where the vast majority of the population are Buddhists, the national version of the instrument included the question "How well are you able to rid yourself of negative feelings through meditation?" in the facet *Negative feelings.* The inclusion of a limited number of culture-specific questions acknowledges that particular aspects of certain facets of quality of life are not universal, and hence enhances the ability of the WHOQOL to address these aspects of quality of life. These questions are in addition to the agreed-upon core questions, however. Furthermore, these "national" questions have to compete with the "global" questions in the analysis of the pilot data to be retained in the instrument.

Response Scale Derivation

The WHOQOL instrument contains response scales concerned with Intensity (Not at all – Extremely), Capacity (Not at all – Completely), Frequency (Never – Always) and Evaluation (Very satisfied – Very dissatisfied; Very good – Very poor). Although endpoints such as "Never" and "Always" are relatively universal, shades of meaning between endpoints (e.g., "sometimes") are more ambiguous, difficult to translate, and subject to cultural variation in their interpretation.

The WHOQOL project utilised a methodology which specifies anchor points for each of the four types of 5-point response scales (Evaluation, Intensity, Capacity and Frequency), and a metric which intermediate descriptors should fit. In brief, this involved translation of the anchor points using the translation methodology outlined below. A list of at least 15 descriptors was then compiled in the language of the field centre for each response scale from dictionaries, a thesaurus, relevant literature, and other psychometric instruments. For each response scale, 20 lay subjects, representative of health care users in the setting, were asked to mark the point on a 100 mm visual analogue scale according to where they thought each descriptor lay in relation to the two anchors. The series of descriptors for a given response scale were presented in random order, and a fresh line was used for each descriptor. The three intermediate descriptors were selected from the means falling in the following ranges: 20 mm – 30 mm, 45 mm – 55 mm, and 70 mm – 80 mm. If several descriptors fell within a given range, the descriptor with the lowest standard deviation was selected. To check on the ordinality of response scales, a small sample of lay respondents was asked to rank order the response scale descriptors for each response scale in a card sort exercise. To check on the comparability of the derived descriptors between centres, a bilingual review process was used. This methodology ensured, first, that response scales are not simply translated from a source language with all the problems associated with this process. Second, it secures a high degree of scalar equivalence between languages. Third, it ensures equidistance between descriptors on the scales.

Piloting of the WHOQOL

A pilot WHOQOL instrument common to all centres was translated into the language of the field centres; it contained 276 core[5] items addressing 30 facets of quality of life, as well as a limited number of national/regional questions. The pilot instrument is being piloted in the period December 1993 to March 1994 on some 250 health care users, with varied levels of quality of life, and 50 well persons in some 12 field centres with the following aim in mind: to refine and reduce the facet structure and reduce the number of questions within facets, while maintaining a common core domain and facet structure across all centres. The ideal is to strike a balance between a minimum number of facets/questions and adequate coverage of the key areas contributing to respondents' quality of life across the cultures included in this phase of work. In the analysis of the pilot data, a mapping procedure that focuses on representativeness and discriminatory power will be used, whereby the association of domains to global questions about quality of life, of facets to domains, and facets to other facets can be examined. On the basis of these data, and importance weightings of individual facets, the facet structure will be refined and reduced. The pooled data will also enable an examination of the possibility that there are several core or primary facets which best summarise quality of life in all centres and certain questions for each of these facets that are reliable and valid in all field centres. A strategy for question selection reflecting "representativeness" (high question-total correlations in the case of the "own" facet) and discriminatory power (low question-total correlations in the case of other facets than the own facet) will be used to select questions that might be present in all national versions of the WHOQOL (for an example of this methodology for question selection see Strelau et al. 1990). Data from individual field centres will then be omitted consecutively to see the effect this has on the refined facet structure. Finally, multi-dimensional scaling will be employed to check further on the structure of the instrument.

The data for each of the project's field centres will then be analyzed separately and the "best" questions will be selected for that centre which define

[5] Those administered in all centres.

each facet most effectively. This analysis will include national questions which will have to compete with the core questions to be retained. After the facet structure and questions have been finalized, it will be possible to use the large data set to examine in a preliminary way the psychometric properties of the instrument, for example, the relationship between facets and the relationship of facets to their respective domains. Reliability will be assessed by examining the internal consistency of questions within each facet and the interchangeability of questions within each facet (split-half). For some facets, however, where more than one concept is being addressed (e.g., *Sensory functions*, seeing and hearing), questions would not be expected to be interchangeable and split-half coefficients would be inappropriate.

The data collected from administering the instrument to a large and diverse group of subjects in each centre will allow for the initial determination of, among other things, its internal consistency and its discriminatory validity.

Reliability, Validity and Responsiveness Studies

After having developed an instrument for each cultural setting, a series of smaller scale studies should be conducted. This will involve the following:

1) clear and homogeneous population(s);
2) longitudinal design, including simultaneous and/or repeated ratings;
3) specific intervention(s) and;
4) parallel use of other national and international instruments with established psychometric properties to assess convergent validity.

From this, the following can be calculated: test-retest reliability, responsiveness to change, cross-validation of the measure and criterion validation, specifically with regard to convergent, discriminant and predictive validity.

Review and Revision

At the end of the developmental phase, the instrument will be reviewed and revised to overcome any difficulties that become apparent. It is possible, for example, that certain facets will be found to be untenable in the light of statistical analyses of the data. For example, facets that show no change across disease and interventions may be of limited value in clinical trials or clinical settings.

Characteristics of the Instrument

The Domains and Facets of Quality of Life

The domains and facets of quality of life for the WHOQOL are shown in Table 1. The way in which these were derived ensures that they are universal, although the questions used to address individual facets and the relative importance of facets in different cultural settings may differ. For example, workers in this area (Olweny 1992) and WHOQOL focus group work suggest that self-esteem is conceived of differently in Western and Eastern cultures, with the "I" being more central to Western conceptions and externally judged esteem within the "We" of one's family or peer group being more important in Eastern cultures. This is indicative of the differing stress on independence and interdependence in these parts of the world. The domains and facets therefore are operationalized so as to be universal, but are flexible enough to allow both universal and culture-specific aspects of the facets to be addressed in the questions asked of respondents in different parts of the world.

Cross-cultural Comparability

Operational equivalence in international health status measures refers to certain psychometric criteria that should be met in each language version of the instrument. This usually pertains to reliability (internal consistency of scales; test-retest), validity (face, consensual, construct, criterion, convergent and discriminant) and responsiveness to change. That is to say two culture/language versions of the instrument should yield comparable reliability, validity and responsiveness data before conclusions can be made about their comparability. These issues are discussed in detail elsewhere in relation to international health status instrument development and will not be repeated here (e.g., Deyo 1984; Hunt 1993; Patrick et al., this volume; Bullinger, this volume).

The "universality" of the WHOQOL arises from:

1) simultaneous development of the instrument in numerous cultural settings;
2) there being a common set of agreed upon facet definitions;
3) a common methodology for question development and selection; and,
4) there being a "global" pool of questions with which any "national" questions have to compete.

In addition, if a number of core facets and questions are found to be reliable and valid across all centres in the analysis of the pilot data, their inclusion will contribute to the universality and cross-cultural comparability of the instrument. Once normative data are available from certain samples of populations, it will be possible to compare in a meaningful way the scores of an individual in one culture with those of an individual in another culture.

Typology of Questions

The focus of the WHOQOL will be a person's perception of life, but there will be separate and distinct enquiry into perceived objective and self-report subjective aspects of quality of life. The questions for both levels are written in general terms and are global self-assessments. Perceived objective questions refer to a person's global evaluations of behaviours, states or capacities, and inform about the individual's assessment of his or her physical and psychological health, level of independence, social relationships and environmental conditions (e.g., "How easily do you get tired?" "How much confidence do you have in yourself?" "How much is your mobility limited?" "Do you get the kind of support from others that you need?"). Self-report subjective questions assess a person's satisfaction/dissatisfaction with his/her behaviour, state or capacity, i.e., to what extent does the person feel that his/her needs and wants are being met, and how much does he/she feel that a problem or difficulty prevents him/her from doing what he/she wants or needs to do (e.g., "How satisfied are you with the energy you have to do what you need to do?" "How much do any feelings of depression bother you?" "How satisfied are you with your ability to communicate with others?"). To assess the validity of the distinction drawn between "perceived objective" and "self-report subjective" questions, two independent raters were asked to assign 36 questions randomly selected from the global question pool to the two categories of question. An inter-rater-reliability of 81% was observed, suggesting substantial reliability in the scheme adopted for the instrument[6]. "Perceived objective" questions tend to be addressed by intensity and frequency questions. "Self-report subjective" questions, on the other hand, tend to comprise primarily evaluation questions.

In addition, standardised "importance questions" have been written for each facet. These are written as "How important to you is ...?" for positively framed facets, and "How important to you is freedom from ...?" for negatively framed facets. These questions will yield information about the relative importance of facets of quality of life in different settings, as well as allow a weighting of individual respondent's scores.

This question typology will enable the WHOQOL to obtain data both about a respondent's perceived objective assessment of facets of his/her life as well as his/her subjective evaluations of these. The instrument will not include questions based on objective measurement of the individual's health and functional status, for instance measuring the quality of sleep, although such data may be used together with the WHOQOL.

Frames of Reference

The frame of reference for the WHOQOL instrument reflects the definition of quality of life adopted for the project. Respondents' quality of life is assessed, therefore, explicitly in relation to their goals, expectations, standards and concerns and implicitly within the context of their culture and value systems in which they live. A time frame of two weeks will be used in piloting the instrument, although different time frames may be necessary for particular

[6] However, for several facets of quality of life the distinction between "perceived objective" and "self-report subjective" questions is less clear, namely *Self esteem, Body image and appearance, Work satisfaction, Positive feelings, and Negative feelings*.

uses of the instrument in subsequent stages of work. For example, in the assessment of quality of life in chronic conditions, such as back pain and arthritis, a longer time frame such as four weeks may be preferable. In the assessment of patients receiving chemotherapy, the treatment cycles should be considered to establish and control for when responsiveness and side effects are anticipated. Furthermore, the perception of time is different in different cultural settings (Sartorius 1987), and this is something that should be explicitly acknowledged in the interpretation of data.

The instructions to respondents state *"Please keep in mind your standards, hopes, pleasures and concerns. We ask that you think about your life in the last two weeks."*

Different Forms of the WHOQOL

Several versions of the WHOQOL will be developed. Because a comprehensive coverage of core areas of quality of life cross-culturally necessitates a relatively long assessment, a shorter version is planned where only primary facets of quality of life are addressed. The short version will have increased utility and will be of particular use in research requiring repeated measures designs, in clinical settings and where respondents have difficulty completing the long version. In addition, interviewer-assisted and interviewer-administered forms of the instrument will be developed for respondents who cannot read or write (for cultural, educational or health reasons).

A quite different form of the instrument could be developed which would be administered by an interviewer who would be free not only to ask set probes but also to develop his/her own probes if necessary to make a rating of certain aspects of quality of life according to criteria set down in a manual and glossary based on the facet definitions as used in the development phase. The interviewer would then be making his or her own interpretation of the responses to make the rating, and for this he/she would need training.

Research using a multi-trait multi-method approach will be directed at establishing the correspondence between these different forms of the instrument.

Uses of the Instrument

It is anticipated that the WHOQOL will have broad-ranging uses. For clinical practice the instrument will assist clinicians in making judgements about the areas in which a patient is most affected by disease and in making treatment decisions. Furthermore, together with other measures, it will allow the assessment of changes over the course of treatment. In some developing countries, where resources for health care may be limited, treatments aimed at improving quality of life through palliation, for example, can be both effective and inexpensive (Olweny 1992).

Furthermore, by increasing the physician's understanding of how disease affects a patient's quality of life, the interaction between patient and doctor will change and improve. This will give more meaning and fulfilment to the work of the doctor and should lead to the patient being provided with more comprehensive health care. Because a comprehensive form of assessment covering different aspects of patients' functioning is being carried out, patients themselves may find their health care more meaningful. Routine use of quality of life instruments such as the WHOQOL will also enhance the recording of patient data, and enable communication of valuable information between professionals.

The WHOQOL will be of considerable use in clinical trials, in establishing baseline scores in a range of areas, and in looking at changes in quality of life over the course of treatment, particularly where disease prognosis is likely to involve only partial recovery or remission and treatment may be more palliative than curative.

For epidemiological research, the WHOQOL will allow detailed quality of life data to be gathered on a particular population. The international epidemiological studies that would be made possible by an instrument such as the WHOQOL will facilitate the understanding of the effects of disease on quality of life, and the development of appropriate health interventions.

In the implementation and planning for new policies it is important that the rationale for and effect of policy changes on the quality of life of people in contact with health services are evaluated. An instrument such as the WHOQOL will allow the planning and monitoring of such changes. That the instrument was developed cross-culturally will allow health care providers, administrators and legislators to be confident that data yielded by work involving the instrument is genuinely sensitive to their setting. Similarly in the periodic review of the completeness and quality of medical services, the WHOQOL will provide an invaluable supplementary appraisal of health care services by yielding a measure of the relationship between the health care service and patients' quality of life, and presenting a measure of patients' perception of the quality and availability of health care.

The WHO initiative to develop a quality of life assessment instrument is linked to other important WHO projects. WHO has projects currently underway on the assessment of different treatments, the development and improvement of the WHO scheme of "impairments, disabilities and handicaps," national guidelines for quality assurance in health care and the monitoring of rehabilitation of psychiatric patients and the subsequent care of the individuals in the community[7]. The WHOQOL project, therefore, is part of a larger drive towards "Health for All," and the promotion of mental, social and physical well-being.

[7] Details of these programmes are available from the Director, Division of Mental Health, World Health Organization, CH-1211 Geneva 27, Switzerland.

Further Language/Culture Versions of the WHOQOL

It is expected that additional centres will want to develop a quality of life instrument besides those in the original study. A manual will be written for the development of instruments in new centres, giving all the procedures to be followed in detail so that any centre can take this up. WHO will continue to provide an international review of questions developed in the centres before adding them to the pool. WHO will also supply the instructions (and possibly software packages, if appropriate) for the analysis of the data collected to develop the local version. The procedure to be followed will be to run focus groups with health care users and health care providers to review the applicability to that culture of the questions in the global pool covering each facet. On the basis of the transcripts of these focus groups, a question-writing panel would be assembled in the new centre to establish whether any additional questions needed to be added to the global question pool for their own cultural setting. If so, the panel should write the questions according to the criteria for WHOQOL questions (Table 2). The questions developed by the new centre would have to be reviewed by WHO, Geneva, to assess if they meet the criteria for WHOQOL questions, before being combined with the global pool of questions. The new centre would then pilot the questions and analyze the data according to the same procedure used in the original study. Thus any new questions proposed by the focus groups and question-writing panel would have to compete with questions in the global pool (questions from all centres) according to psychometric criteria to be included. The new centre would then also be expected to set up studies in which the reliability, validity and sensitivity of the instrument were established.

In addition, WHO aims to facilitate the establishment of quality of life assessment training centres within countries. These would be centres of excellence where people would receive training in quality of life assessment. This training would focus on the theoretical background of quality of life, the assessment of quality of life, the evaluation of quality of life measures and the implementation of quality of life measures in health care settings. These centres would further aim to coordinate quality of life research involving the WHOQOL and provide technical assistance to those using the instrument.

Population-Specific Modules of the WHOQOL

The core instrument will be developed initially. A number of specific WHOQOL modules will be developed later, as add-on modules to the core instrument, for assessing people with a particular disease or in circumstances in which the core module does not provide sufficient detail. WHO has identified five priority areas for module development: 1) persons suffering from chronic diseases (e.g., epilepsy, arthritis, cancer, AIDS, diabetes); 2) caregivers of the ill or disabled (e.g., a person taking care of a terminally sick patient); 3) persons living in highly stressful situations (e.g. elderly people living in poorly run institutions, refugees in camps); 4) persons with difficulty communicating (e.g., persons with severe learning disabilities); and 5) children. The methodology for the development of modules is detailed elsewhere (WHO, 1993 c), but includes the same iterative process of input from health professionals and quality of life researchers from around the world, cross-cultural lay review (through the use of focus groups), and international expert review. The methodology also states that any module should be developed simultaneously in at least three culturally diverse centres.

Summary

In conclusion, WHO's commitment to the development of a quality of life assessment arises from the lack of any genuinely international instruments that can be meaningfully used in both developed and developing world countries to measure the individual's subjective view of the impact of disease and impairment on his/her life. Work on this project restates WHO's commitment to a holistic view of health, and the need for a humanistic element in health care that goes beyond the eradication of symptoms and disease. The WHOQOL has been designed as a generic instrument for the assessment of both positive and negative aspects of quality of life. It will be a multilingual and multidimensional profile yielding quality of life scores in six domains and some 20 to 30 facets of quality of life. This chapter outlines the characteristics of the WHOQOL, as well as the steps employed in its development.

References

Bergner M, Bobbitt, RA, Carter WB et al. (1981) The Sickness Impact Profile: Development and final revision of a health status measure. Med Care 19:787–805

Bowling A (1991) Measuring health: a review of quality of life measurement scales. Philadelphia: Open University Press

Deyo R (1984) Pitfalls in measuring the health status of Mexican Americans: Comparative validity of the English and Spanish Sickness Impact Profile. Am J Public Health 74:569–573

Fallowfield L (1990) The quality of life: the missing measurement in health care. Souvenir Press

Gerin P, Dazord A, Boissel J, Chifflet R (1992) Quality of life assessment in therapeutic trials: Rationale for and presentation of a more appropriate instrument. Fund Clin Pharmacol 6:263–276

Hunt SM (1993) Cross-cultural comparability of quality of life measures. Drug Info J 27:395–400

Hunt SM, McKenna, SP, McEwan J (1989) The Nottingham Health Profile. Users Manual. Revised edition

McDowell I, Newell C (1987) Measuring health: a guide to rating scales and questionnaires. New York: Oxford University Press

Morgan DL (1988) Focus groups as qualitative research. Qual Res Meth Series 16: Sage
Olweny CLM (1992) Quality of life in developing countries. J Palliative Care 8:25–30
Patrick DL, Erikson P (1993) Health status and health policy: allocating resources to health care. Oxford University Press, New York
Quality of Life Bibliography and Indexes (1990) Med Care 28(Supplement):DS1–DS77
Sartorius N (1987) Cross-cultural comparisons of data about quality of life: A sample of issues. In: Aaronson NK, Beckman J (eds) The quality of life of cancer patients. New York, Raven Press
Sartorius N (1988) Cross-cultural and international collaboration in mental health research and action: Experience from the mental health programme of the World Health Organization. In: Janson R, Perris C (eds) Acta Scand Psychiat 78 (Supplement 344):71–74
Strelau J, Angleitner A, Bantelmann J, Ruch W (1990) The Strelau Temperament Inventory-Revised (STI-R): Theoretical considerations and scale development. Eur J Personality 4:209–235
Walker SR, Rosser RM (eds) (1993) Quality of life assessment: key issues in the 1990's. Lancaster, UK: Kluwer Academic Publishers
Ware JE, Snow KK, Kosinski M, Gandek B (1993) SF-36 Health Survey: manual and interpretation guide. New England Medical Center, MA, USA
World Bank (1993) World Development Report: investing in Health. New York: Oxford University Press
World Health Organization (1991). World Health Statistics Annual. Geneva: WHO
World Health Organization (1992a). Meeting on Quality of Life. Geneva: WHO (MNH/PSF/92.2)
World Health Organization (1992b) Report of the Meeting of Investigators on Quality of Life. Geneva: WHO (MNH/PSF/92.6)
World Health Organization (1992c) WHOQOL Focus group Moderator Training. Geneva: WHO (MNH/PSF/92.9)
World Health Organization (1993a) Report of WHOQOL Focus Group Work. Geneva: WHO (MNH/PSF/93.4)
World Health Organization (1993b) Report of WHO/IPSEN Foundation Joint Meeting on Quality of Life Assessment. Geneva. WHO (MNH/PSF/93.5)
World Health Organization (1993c) WHOQOL Study Protocol. Geneva: WHO (MNH/PSF/93.9)
The WHOQOL Group (1993) Study protocol for the World Health Organization project to develop a Quality of Life assessment instrument (WHOQOL). Qual Life Res 2:153–159

Perspectives on Quality of Life

The Relationship Between Health Economics and Health-Related Quality of Life

J.A. Fox-Rushby

Summary

Health economics has benefitted from, and contributed towards, the field of health-related quality of life (HRQL). This chapter describes the framework of economic evaluation and shows where, and why, measures of HRQL are used. The main contribution of health economics has occurred in the area of valuation, and a range of valuation techniques is presented. Increased demand for economic evaluations by central level decision-makers all over the world has resulted in the development of league tables of cost-effectiveness and the raising of justifiable questions regarding international comparability of costs and HRQL.

Introduction

One of the basic problems facing decision-makers in the health sector is how to spend scarce resources in the face of competing needs. The absence of a freely functioning price system requires a careful consideration of the costs and consequences of alternative interventions. This basic framework for *aiding* decision-making can be applied at the micro level (choosing one of two treatments for the same condition) or at a broader level (choosing how to allocate the whole health service budget or how much to allocate to the health sector versus other sectors).

The importance of economic evaluation within the health sector has been heightened in the last few years at both levels. The Commonwealth of Australia (1990) and the Ontario Ministry of Health (1991) have issued guidelines to encourage a standardised approach to economic evaluation. The rise in the number of economic evaluations can be attributed to an era of competition, the use of economic evaluations by pharmaceutical companies as a marketing tool, advances in the methodology itself and the use of economic evaluation at macro levels of decision-making.

At micro and macro levels of decision-making in health care, the assessment of health-related quality of life (HRQL) is an integral part of health economics. First, health economics is a *user* of HRQL measurement instruments and secondly, health economics has been instrumental in *developing* the area of

J. Orley, W. Kuyken (Eds.)
Quality of Life Assessment:
International Perspectives

HRQL. This chapter is divided into three sections. The first outlines the range of economic evaluations and describes the type of question each seeks to address. The second part describes the symbiotic relationship of health economics and HRQL and the final section reviews some general issues of practice, including league tables and international assessment of HRQL.

The Framework of Economic Evaluation

Economic evaluation is designed specifically to promote efficiency and poses questions like, "Are limited resources used in the best possible ways?" It has been defined as "the comparative analysis of alternative courses of action in terms of both their costs and consequences" (Drummond et al. 1987). Therefore the two most important characteristics are dealing with inputs and outputs as well as having at least two alternatives for comparison. The analysis of efficiency is founded within the theory of welfare economics, which promotes two concepts of efficiency: productive[1] or allocative[2] efficiency. Table 1 shows the different types of economic evaluation. The clear difference between the methods is in the measurement (and valuation) of consequences. A less obvious difference is the type of questions posed and notion of efficiency investigated.

Cost minimisation analysis (CMA) assesses the cheapest of two options available. Most importantly this method assumes (from epidemiological findings or published clinical evidence) that each option has an identical outcome. The advantage is that it is a relatively quick form of analysis but often it is hampered by the unreliability of assuming that consequences are equal.

Cost effectiveness analysis (CEA) can be used in one of two situations:

1) when interventions achieve a given outcome at least cost;
2) when interventions maximise effectiveness subject to a fixed budget constraint.[3]

Effectiveness can be measured in "natural" units, such as unit of blood pressure reduction, or, more broadly, life years gained. The advantage of CEA is that the analysis of technical efficiency can be applied to a range of measures from clinical outcomes to assessment of activities of daily living and impact

[1] Productive (or technical) efficiency is the achievement of the maximum obtainable output of *x* given the output of *y*, or vice versa. This corresponds to production being *on* the production possibility frontier, i.e., the maximum possible production is achieved. This analysis assumes all factors of production are fully employed. Productive efficiency is analysed subject to a budget constraint.

[2] Productive efficiency is a necessary, but not sufficient-condition for allocative efficiency. Allocative efficiency (Pareto Optimality) exists when "it is no longer possible to so reallocate resources as to increase the economic welfare of one individual except at the expense of another (Laidler, 1981).

[3] Some of the methodological concerns are discussed in Birch and Gafni (1992).

Table 1. Measurement of costs and consequences in economic evaluation

Type of study	Measurement/ valuation of costs in both alternatives	Identification of consequences	Measurement/ valuation of consequences
Cost-minimisation analysis	Dollars	Identical in all respects	None
Cost-effectiveness analysis	Dollars	Single effect of interest, common to both alternatives, but achieved to different degrees	Natural units (e.g., life-years gained, disability days saved, points of blood pressure reduction, etc.)
Cost-benefit analysis	Dollars	Single or multiple effects, not necessarily common to both alternatives, and common effects may be achieved to different degrees by the alternatives	Dollars
Cost-utility analysis	Dollars	Single or multiple effects, not necessarily common to both alternatives, and common effects may be achieved to different degrees by the alternatives	Healthy days or (more often) quality adjusted life-years

Source: Drummond et al. (1987)

on health status. The narrower the measure of consequences, the smaller the degree of comparability with interventions outside a particular field but the more closely any measured change can be related to the intervention. Medical interventions can affect a whole variety of aspects of health, each of which is measurable by different instruments.[4] CEA, however, is designed only to compare interventions which have the same types of outcome; thus interventions with different outcomes cannot be compared.

Cost benefit analysis (CBA) is the only method available aimed at assessing allocative efficiency. In this case both costs and consequences are valued in monetary terms. This ensures that results and comparisons do not have to be

[4] See Croog et al. (1986) and Bombardier et al. (1986) who applied "batteries of tests of effectiveness."

limited to one sector. If the net benefit exceeds zero,[5] an intervention is preferred. Translating effects into money values is a difficult and contentious, though not necessarily insurmountable, task.

Cost utility analysis (CUA) developed from the need to compare health programmes with different outcomes. The consequences of an intervention are assessed not in physical units, but in utilities. The objective of utilities is to represent social preferences for health outcomes. Even though CUA incorporates issues of consumption, it remains an assessment of technical efficiency because it is tied to fixed budget constraints.

The principal theoretical differences between these four methods are the assessment of consequences and level of efficiency sought. CMA, CEA and CUA implicitly assume the health objectives of an intervention are worthwhile whereas CBA, in theory, allows judgement of the health objectives per se. Practically, however, the degree of constraints imposed by data requirements also differs dramatically, with CBA facing the largest task.

HRQL and Health Economics

Drummond et al. (1987) recommended undertaking three steps in investigation of costs and consequences in economic evaluation: identification, measurement and valuation. Applying the latter two categories to HRQL highlights the symbiotic nature of health economics and HRQL assessment.

Contribution of HRQL Assessment to Health Economics

The development of *measures* of HRQL has catapulted a whole range of effects into the realm of economic evaluation. Where economic evaluations were once restricted to measuring costs against proxy indicators or partial indicators of effect (e.g., lives saved), they can now encompass the whole spectrum of measured changes. Therefore economic evaluation can be applied to clinical through to functional assessment and generic measures of health. Advances in the methodological rigour of outcome assessment have increased the confidence attached to the results of economic evaluations. The range of outcome measures developed has allowed CEA to remain a flexible tool which can be focused on the question at hand. Therefore, CEA can be applied to assess the efficiency of two alternative treatments designed to reduce breathlessness on exertion or to evaluate the efficiency of two interventions for very different diseases in terms of their effects on HRQL.

---

[5] The decision rule is:

$(B_A - C_A) - (B_B - C_B) > 0$

OR, $(B_A - B_B) - (C_A - C_B) > 0$

where B = Benefits, C = Costs, $_{A/B}$ = Intervention $_A$ or $_B$.

The main dichotomy presented in the field of measuring HRQL is whether to use disease-specific or generic measures of HRQL. Disease-specific measures concentrate on "the symptoms, complaints, disabilities and disruptions in life that are specific to the clinical condition under study" (Williams and Wood-Dauphinee 1989). Clinicians more frequently request disease-specific measures than generic measures in the context of clinical trials because of the ability to tailor the questionnaire to specific needs. The many disease-specific measures available cover both a wide range of disease and areas of HRQL. Disease-specific instruments are more responsive than generic measures to within-patient change over time, although this is at the expense of reliability (Guyatt et al. 1987). Measured change is also easier to interpret given that the measures are more closely related to clinical assessments of disease activity (Patrick and Deyo 1989). Finally, disease-specific measures "may enjoy the advantage of ease in administration, acceptability, cost and simplicity in scoring precisely because they are designed for application in clinical settings" (Patrick and Deyo 1989). The disadvantage is that results cannot be compared with other disease groups.

Generic instruments differ in that they are "applicable in a wide variety of populations because they cover the complete spectrum of function, disability and distress that is relevant to quality of life" (Guyatt et al. 1989) and can be produced as profiles or indices. Profiles do not produce a single "score" for health but a "picture" of an individual's health. The disadvantage with health profiles is that no single index is produced, so a definitive answer is not always possible in the comparison of two therapies and thus profiles cannot be used in broad resource allocation decisions. However, the advantage is that, as the dimensions of health included are more numerous than in a global index, sensitivity is greater. The majority of profiles have been developed in North America: McMaster Health Index Questionnaire (Chambers et al. 1982), Sickness Impact Profile (SIP)[6] (Bergner et al. 1981), and the SF-36 (Ware and Sherbourne 1992). The Nottingham Health Profile (Hunt et al. 1986) is the only general health profile developed in the UK.

There are several advantages to using generic measures. The most important is comparability of results across different populations and disease groups. There has been a concerted effort in producing valid and reliable scales which has encouraged their widespread use, particularly of the SIP. Widespread use has the added advantage of population norms often being available. The disadvantages associated with generic measures are, first, that they may be insensitive to marginal changes in clinical trials. Second, the end points of scales are often arbitrary, so that 0 does not indicate zero health and 100 is not equal to perfect health. Third, there is a particular inability to differentiate at the points of extreme health or ill health although, to some extent, the SF-36 attempts to overcome this problem by asking about positive aspects of health (Brazier et al. 1992).

---

[6] The SIP is the only profile which can also produce a single score.

The Contribution of Health Economics to HRQL Assessment

It is in the area of valuation that health economics has had the greatest contribution to the development of HRQL assessment. Valuation sets out to "estimate the worth, desirability and utility of a thing, or the qualities on which these depend" (Concise Oxford Dictionary, 1990). Research has centred on both non-monetary and monetary valuation methods, with the majority of research in the former area. Thus, valuation techniques have most often been applied to CUA rather than CBA. An example of a question involving valuation would be: given an increase in mobility from being able to walk with crutches to being able to walk with the aid of a walking stick, how desirable is that change? The advantage of pursuing HRQL beyond the stage of measurement to valuation is that very different characteristics of HRQL can be valued on a single scale and therefore be made comparable.

Drummond et al. (1987) point to three methods available for establishing utility values: judgement, values from the literature or values from measurements on a sample of subjects. The first approach is the simplest and quickest and, using a detailed sensitivity analysis, could easily examine the robustness of utility values. Those values subject to significant variation under sensitivity analysis could also be used as a means of directing future work on providing values. In terms of the second approach, whilst there is a growing literature available with reference points for utilities for some specific health states, it is not a large literature. This reduces the likelihood of matching health state values already valued with the particular needs of any one evaluation. The third method, measurement, is generally the most accurate and is necessary either where values are shown to be sensitive to varied assumptions or where they are not available.

Given the need to measure utilities attached to a particular health state, there are two options open in the measurement approach: first, to ask patients with the health state in question to value their utility for it or, second, to write a description of the health state (a scenario) and ask either a "lay" person or "expert" to place their value on the state. The advantage of the first approach is that respondents would be able to understand how they felt, which is more difficult in a hypothetical situation. However, individuals only experience a small number of conditions. The use of scenarios is advantageous in allowing any one individual to value a number of different health states. In addition to this, the ability to reflect very diverse characteristics of health states and other factors, such as age, can be introduced (Buxton and Ashby 1988). For these reasons, scenarios have usually been the preferred approach. Once a particular set of scenarios have been agreed upon, there are a variety of methods available to elicit preferences: standard gamble (SG), time trade-off (TTO), rating scales, equivalence technique, magnitude estimation and willingness-to-pay (WTP).

The strength of the SG is its base in the axioms of expected utility theory and it is the classic method used for measuring cardinal preferences[7] which

[7] (Footnote see page 67)

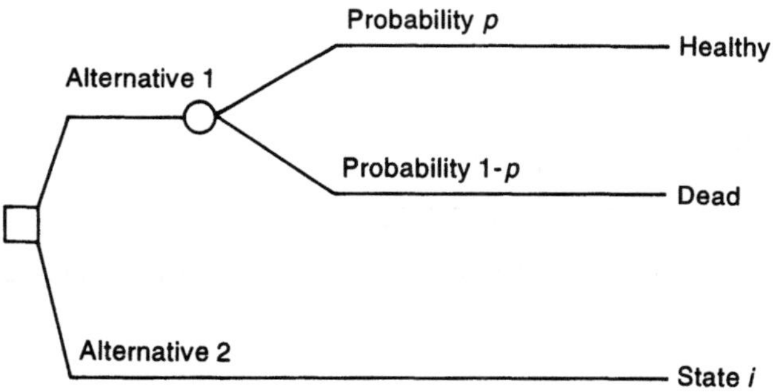

Fig. 1. Standard Gamble for a Chronic Health State Preferred to Death. Source: Torrance (1986)

explicitly accounts for uncertainty. Subjects are asked to choose between a certain outcome of state *i* for time *t* years or a chance (p) of either health for *t* years and immediate death ($1-p$). The probability (p) is varied to determine the maximum risk of death the person would accept until the point of indifference is reached. Figure 1 depicts the gamble. The point of indifference is affected by a number of factors. If the health state is perceived as particularly undesirable, the individual is more likely to accept a higher probability of death. Therefore if $p = 0.8$, the value attached to the health state would be $1-0.8 = 0.2$. However, the values assigned by standard gamble are not *only* affected by the perceived severity of health state. This particular technique is contaminated by two aversions: to gambling itself and risk. Respondents have also found it difficult to cope with probabilities (Torrance 1986), so that the technique is best suited to interviews, which tend to take a long time.

The TTO technique was developed by Torrance et al. (1972) specifically for use in health care. As respondents found probabilities difficult to understand in the SG technique, probabilities were excluded and thus it became a simpler technique to explain and understand. Figure 2 is a graphic representation of the choices offered using this technique. The first alternative offers an individual a particular outcome for a specified length of time (t) followed by death. The second alternative offers a higher HRQL for a shorter length of time (x). This time is varied until the respondent is indifferent between the two alternatives. The indirect preference value is given by x/t[8]. The prediction from this technique is that the worse a health state is perceived to be, the more time a

[7] Ordinal preferences are a ranked set of preferences. Cardinal preferences differ in that an attempt is made to ascertain the distance between one category and another. Cardinal scales can be of two types, interval or ratio. Interval scales incorporate a procedure for equating the intervals between the ranks. Ratio scales have true zero points so that it is possible to deal with proportions.

[8] As Torrance (1986) explained, "One difficulty which has arisen in practice is that, although the method imposes an upper limit of 1.0 on states of health preferred to death, it imposes no comparable lower limit on states dispreferred to death."

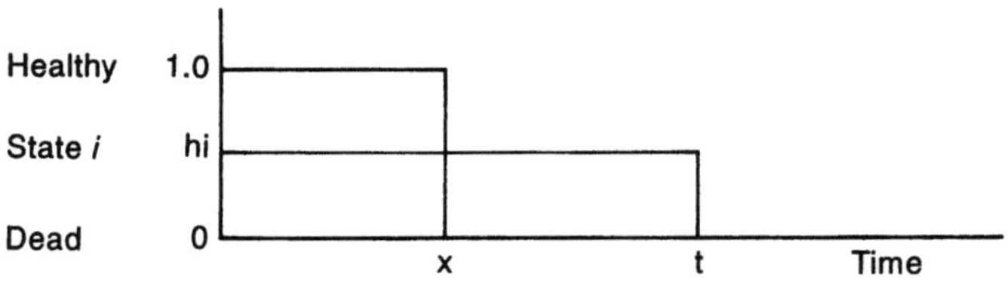

Fig. 2. Time Trade-Off for a Chronic Health State Preferred to Death. Source: Torrance (1986)

person would be willing to give up to life in "perfect health." TTO is not derived from the axioms of expected utility theory and requires the additional assumption that the respondent's utility function for additional healthy years be linear with time, which has been criticised (Feeney and Torrance 1988).

Rating scales require subjects to rate health states on a scale with two defined end points. A good example of this is that developed by the EuroQol Group (1990), where subjects are asked to place descriptions of different health states on a scale from 0–100 (labelled worst imaginable health state to best imaginable health state) and in relation to each other. Rating scales can be used to measure preferences for both chronic and temporary health states. The advantages of rating scales are their practicality because they are efficient and easy to use. Second, their applicability to laboratory situations, surveys, interviews or self-completed questionnaires explains their extensive use. The drawbacks to this approach are, first, it has no *theoretical* basis and, secondly, it is subject to contextual effects such as response spreading[9].

The remaining methods for assessing strength of preferences – magnitude estimation, equivalence technique and contingent valuation – have been the focus of far less research (Froberg and Kane 1989). Magnitude estimation, which was used by Rosser and Kind (1978) and Gudex et al. (Gudex et al. 1993), poses the following type of question, "How many times worse is state A compared with state B?" The equivalence technique, which is similar, identifies the respondent's point of indifference between keeping two different groups of people alive by varying the numbers in the groups. It involves direct interpersonal comparison of utility and this is considered offensive by some. The approach is currently being pursued by Nord (1992).

As with methods for non-monetary valuation, there are a variety of possible ways to estimate the monetary valuation of the consequences of health care interventions[10]. Contingent valuation via expressed preferences[11] has the most

[9] Response spreading is caused by a respondent's desire to use each category on a scale equally often.

[10] This includes the human capital (or livelihood) approach, expenditure on insurance, court awards, implicit public sector valuation and contingent valuation.

[11] Expressed preferences is the direct questioning of individuals about their own valuations as opposed to "revealed" preferences (the observation of actual choices where risk has been traded off against income).

cogent theoretical base and offers the greatest potential for analysis and understanding of factors affecting preferences (Fox-Rushby 1993). Contingent valuation is centred in consumer surplus[12], the estimation of which is required in order to value the benefits of a publicly provided, non-marketed good such as health care. An example of a question asked would be, "What is the maximum (minimum) you would be willing to pay (accept) for an increase (decrease) in [a specified charge in health status]?"[13] The advantage is that consequences can be compared directly with costs and with interventions outside the health sector. However, the disadvantages are that ability to pay affects valuations and that little is known about the psychometric properties of willingness-to-pay/receive valuations (Mulley 1989).

The techniques described so far have been used to assign utility values to health states. However, the utility values have also been applied in the context of relative preferences for quality *and* quantity of life. "Quality adjusted" life years (QALYs) combine quality and quantity of HRQL in one dimension (Williams 1984). The most common method of creating this index is a simple multiplication of life years and the utility attached to those years in particular states of health. The assumption that the value given to any health state is independent of the time spent in it has been criticised by Loomes and McKenzie (1989) and Buxton (1992). Mehrez and Gafni (1989) have pursued the criticisms further in their presentation of the healthy life year equivalents (HYEs). The main difference is that HYEs do not assume inter-temporal additive separability whereas QALYs do. However, whether HYEs is a superior approach has not been substantiated empirically (Culyer and Wagstaff 1992).

The development of tools to value changes in HRQL have been pursued from desires for generalisability, in order to inform a rational and explicit resource allocation process. However, it should be recognised that the area is still evolving as various difficulties are confronted. These include the lack of precision of single measurements of utility, the need for skilled people for labour-intensive interviews and the difficulty of universally applying such complex procedures (Feeny and Torrance 1988).

The Use of Economic Evaluation and Health-related Quality of Life in Policy Making

The majority of work in economic evaluation of health interventions has been conducted under CEA (Backhouse et al. 1992). Gerard (1992) was able to identify only 51 studies of CUA, and there are far fewer studies of CBA in health

---

[12] Consumer surplus is the difference between the amount a consumer is willing to pay for a good/service and the amount she/he actually pays for it. Increments in consumer surplus are equated with increases in consumer welfare (Mishan 1971).

[13] This is the compensating variation in income which is the variation in income at new prices necessary to attain the original indifference curve.

care using WTP by expressed preferences as a method for valuing consequences (Robinson 1993). Therefore the measurement of HRQL forms the largest body or work in assessing consequences.

The increasing demand for full economic evaluations using generic measures of HRQL has risen not only in countries where HRQL instruments have been developed, but across the world. Coupled with interest in cross-cultural comparisons (Hunt 1986) and norms (Aaronson et al. 1992) as well as the desire to highlight inequalities in health between cultural groups (Ahmed et al. 1989), it is understandable that the demand for culturally applicable measures of generic HRQL has risen. There have been two responses to this demand; first to translate, test and adapt existing measures in different countries and secondly, to develop an international instrument at the outset. As Alonso et al. (1990) stated, developing a new measure is a time-consuming and complex task and this is the prime reason for the translation and adaptation of existing instruments. This approach has been adopted for the Nottingham Health Profile (Hunt et al. 1991), SIP (Hendricson et al. 1989) and SF-36 (Aaronson et al. 1992; Brazier et al. 1992) and, with this experience, recommendations are now appearing to encourage a standardised, higher quality approach to this process. The second approach has been adopted by the WHOQOL (Orley 1992) and EuroQol (1990). The disadvantage of the first approach is that the dimensions of HRQL that are included are not taken from definitions of health and illness of the new population; therefore it is more likely that a relevant dimension will be overlooked. To date, the only internationally developed instrument able to produce an index is the EuroQol instrument.

The impact in policy making of individual economic evaluations of interventions for specific diseases and populations is gradually being considered (Alban 1987; Davies et al. 1993; Gerard 1992). The types of questions raised of micro studies have centred on the quality of the economic evaluation, methods of dissemination, source of funds for study and purpose of evaluation. Gerard (1992) showed that only 50% of researchers "were aware of any influence that the results had." This may be related to another finding that "only one third of all studies had informing government policy or decision-making as their primary objective" (Davies et al. 1993). Whilst these results are surprising, it is likely that influence will increase as future purchasers and providers of health interventions will be required to assess cost-effectiveness of health interventions as well as being given more guidance on how to conduct economic evaluations (Drummond 1992)[14].

The impact of economic evaluation at broader levels of decision-making has been influenced by presentation of "league tables" of cost-effectiveness. A discursive article by Williams (1984) presented a "league table" of comparative cost/QALY gained for a variety of health interventions. Recently "league tables" have been extended and applied by national level decision-makers in the

[14] WHO publishes a number of manuals designed to instruct programme managers in the science and art of conducting economic evaluations. Drummond et al. (1987) is one of the commonly used forms of instruction in developed countries.

United States as a method for allocating resources (Health Services Commission 1991) and circulated to health authorities in the United Kingdom to encourage cost-effective purchasing of health care. Jamison et al. (1993) have reviewed the cost-effectiveness of a large range of interventions relating to developing countries and the World Development Report (1993) has propounded the use of "league tables"[15] at international and national levels. The aim is to influence bilateral and multilateral aid agencies, non-governmental organisations and national governments in their decisions on funding health care.

As Drummond et al. (1993) wrote, "the mere act of assembling data on a range of interventions gives greater prominence to the cost-effectiveness data than does the reporting of the studies individually." The interpretation of these tables is crucial and has stimulated both critical and constructive debate (Drummond et al. 1993; Gerard and Mooney 1993). Simple presentations of (seemingly comparable) costs and QALYs gained mask many differences, such as methods used for calculating QALYs, types of costs counted and choice of alternatives considered. In addition, an implicit assumption is that the rankings are transferable to different health care contexts and different periods of time. This is unlikely to be the case. It is important to consider the applicability of results to "local" circumstances in terms of costs and consequences. The cross-cultural research on HRQL will have an important role in this debate. The interesting finding from the EuroQol Group (1990) was that the absolute and relative values placed on a range of health states in three European countries were closely related, indicating a broad agreement. It will be interesting to see whether this finding holds outside the European context[16].

Conclusions

The majority of applications of economic evaluation have been CEA. The types of measures of health-related quality of life used within these analyses have included disease-specific and generic measures. The aim is usually to compare two specific forms of intervention for the purpose of informing local and national decisions. The flexibility of CEA as a tool for assessing the efficiency of medical interventions has increased with the advent of a wider range of outcome measures.

The role economics has played in the development of the field of HRQL has been greatest in the area of valuation, and the fields of consumer surplus and

[15] The World Development Report (1993) uses cost per DALY (disability adjusted life year) rather than cost per QALY. The DALY does not take any account of individual preferences and therefore does not compare with other league tables of CUA. It uses a measure of effect rather than utility.

[16] There is little evidence of the cultural applicability of the existing non-monetary methods of assessing utility. Tan-Torres (1990) showed evidence of the standard gamble failing in the Philippines due to radically different verbal expressions of risk and certainty.

utility theory have provided theoretical bases from which to undertake empirical work. The drive for comparability of information at central levels of decision-making has increased the desire for generic indices of HRQL. As a result, there is a growing use of CUA and CBA. Methodological advances in utility assessment using principles from economics have enabled new instruments to "enter the market," and cost/QALY league tables have become increasingly common. There have been important and pertinent criticisms of the construction of league tables. First, more information should be provided to ensure that proper comparisons allow for differences in measuring and valuing HRQL, costs, time periods, scale of operations, etc. Secondly, whilst the *methods* may be comparable, results may not be directly transferable into different settings.

The future will, hopefully, unfurl a more constructive debate on how to relate league tables to different settings and on the context to which it is cost effective to create national league tables and develop or adapt culturally applicable measures of HRQL. The development by the EuroQol group to assess the valuation of specific health states in different countries is the only attempt, so far, to address issues of international valuation.

Finally, a summary measure of efficiency is only one factor to take into account in the decision-making. First, factors affecting efficiency should be considered (Berman 1982) and, second, issues of equity are an integral consideration in the development of health policy. Thus economic evaluation can, and should, present only a *partial* set of information to decision-makers; it is an aid to, not a substitute for, decision-making.

Acknowledgements

Julia Fox-Rushby is a member of the Health Economics and Financing Programme, supported by the Overseas Development Administration (ODA). The author would also like to thank Clare Gudex, Anne Mills, Charles Normand and Liz Butters for helpful comments. However, the views in this paper are attributable to the author alone.

References

Aaronson N, Acquadro C, Alonso J, Apolone G, Bucquet D, Bullinger M, Bungay K, Fukuhara S, Gandek B, Keller S, Razavi D, Sanson-Fisher R, Sullivan M, Wood-Dauphinee S, Wagner A, Ware J (1992) International quality of life assessment (IQOLA) project. Quality Life Res 1:349–351

Ahmed W, Kernohan E, Baker M (1989) Cross-cultural use of socio-medical indicators in British Asians. Health Pol 13:95–102

Alban A (1987) Economic appraisal: what is the use revisited. Paper presented at the Eighth Nordic Health Economists' Study Group

Alonso J, Anto JM, Moreno C (1990) Spanish version of the Nottingham Health Profile: translation and preliminary validity Am J Public Health 80:6:704–708

Backhouse M, Backhouse R, Edey S (1992) Economic evaluation bibliography. Health Econ 1 (suppl):1–236
Bergner M, Bobbitt RA, Carter WB, Gilson BS (1981) The Sickness Impact Profile: Development and final revision of a health status measure. Med Care 19:785–805
Berman P (1982) Selective primary health care: Is efficient sufficient? Social Sci Med 16:1056
Birch S, Gafni A (1992) Cost-Effectiveness/Utility Analyses: Do current decision rules lead us to where we want to be? J Health Econ 11:279–296
Bombardier C, Ware J, Russel IJ, Laison M, Chalmers A, Leighton-Read (1986) Auranofin in therapy and quality of life of patients with rheumatoid arthritis. Am J Med 81:565–578
Brazier J, Harper R, Jones N, Cathain A, Usherwood T, Westlake L (1992) Validation of the SF-36 Health Survey Questionnaire: New outcome measure for primary care. Brit Med J 305:6346, 160–164
Buxton M (1992) Uncertainties with QALYs and possible improvements. In: Hopkins A (ed) Different measures of the quality of life and the uses to which they may be put. Royal College of Physicians, London, UK
Buxton M, Ashby J (1988) The Time Trade-Off approach to health state valuation. In: Teeling-Smith G (ed) Measuring health: A practical approach. John Wiley, Chichester
Chambers LW, MacDonald LA, Tugwell P, Buchanan W, Kraag G (1982) The McMaster Health Index Questionnaire as a measure of quality of life for patients with rheumatoid arthritis. J Rheumatol 9:780–784
Commonwealth of Australia (1990) Guidelines for preparation of submissions to the Pharmaceutical Benefits Advisory Committee: including submissions involving economic analyses. Woden (ACT) Department of Health, Housing and Community Services
Croog SH, Levine S, Testa M, Brown B, Bulpitt C, Jenkins D, Klerman G, Williams G (1986) The effect of anti-hypertensive therapy on the quality of life. New Engl Med J 26:1657–1665
Culyer A, Wagstaff A (1992) QALYs versus HYEs: a theoretical exposition. Centre for Health Economics Discussion Paper No. 99. University of York, UK
Davies L, Coyle D, Drummond M (1993) Current status of economic appraisal of health technology in the European Community: Report of the network. Paper presented to International Society of Technology Assessment in Health Care, Sorrento
Drummond M (1992) Cost-effectiveness guidelines for reimbursement of pharmaceuticals: Is economic evaluation ready for its enhanced status? Health Econ 1:85–92
Drummond M, Stoddart G, Torrance G (1987) Methods for the economic evaluation of health care programmes. Oxford Medical Publications, Oxford University Press
Drummond M, Torrance G, Mason J (1993) Cost-effectiveness league tables: more harm than good? Social Sci Med 37:1:33–40
EuroQol Group (1990) EuroQol: A new facility for the measurement of health related quality of life. Health Pol 16:199–208
Feeny D, Torrance GW (1988) Incorporating utility based quality of life assessment measures in clinical trials: Two examples. McMaster University Working Papers
Fox-Rushby J (1993) The measurement and valuation of health related quality of life: The case of differing pacing modalities. Doctoral Thesis, Brunel University
Froberg D, Kane K (1989) Methodology for health state preferences: Part 4 J Clin Epidemiol 22:675–685
Gerard K (1992) Cost Utility Analysis: A policy makers guide to the state of the art. Health Pol 21:3:249–280
Gerard K, Mooney G (1993) QALY league tables: handle with care. Health Econ 2:59–64
Gudex C, Kind P, van Dalen H, Durand M, Morris J, Williams A (1993) Comparing scaling methods for health state valuations – Rosser revisited. Centre for Health Economics Discussion Paper No 107, York University
Guyatt G, Walter S, Norman G (1987) Measuring Change over time: assessing the usefulness of evaluative instruments. J Chronic Diseases 38:517–524

Guyatt G, van Zanten S, Feeny D, Patrick D (1989) Measuring quality of life in clinical trials. J Chronic Diseases 40:171–178

Health Services Commission (1991) The Prioritised Health Services List. Salern: HSC, USA

Hendricson W, Russell I, Prihoda T, Jacobson J, Rogan A, Bishop G (1989) An Approach to developing a valid Spanish language translation of a health-status questionnaire. Med Care 27:10:959–966

Hunt S (1986) Cross cultural issues in the use of socio-medical indicators. Health Pol 6:149–158

Hunt SM, McEwen S, McKenna SP (1986) Measuring Health Status. Croom Helm, London

Hunt S, Alonso J, Bucquet D, Niero M, Wiklund I, McKenna S (1991) Cross-cultural adaptation of health measures. Health Pol 19:33–44

Jamison D, Mosley W, Measham A, Bobadilla J (eds) (1993) Disease control priorities in developing countries. Oxford Medical Publications, Oxford

Laidler D (1981) Introduction to microeconomics. Philip Allan Publishers, Oxford

Loomes G, McKenzie L (1989) The use of QALYs in health care decision making. Social Sci Med 28:4:299–308

Mehrez A, Gafni A (1989) Quality Adjusted Life Years, utility theory and health-years equivalents. Med Decision Making 9:142–149

Mishan EJ (1971) Cost-Benefit Analysis. Unwin University Books, UK

Mulley AG (1989) Assessing patient's utilities: Can the end justify the means? Med Care 27:5269–5281

Nord E (1992) An alternative to QALYs: The saved young life equivalent (SAVE) Brit Med J 305:875–877

Ontario Ministry of Health (1991) Guidelines for preparation of economic analysis to be included in submission to Drug Programs Branch for listing in the Ontario Drug Benefit Formulary/Comparative Drug Index. Toronto, Ministry of Health

Orley J (1992) News from the World Health Organisation. Quality Life Res 1:277

Patrick D, Deyo R (1989) Generic and disease specific measures in assessing health status and quality of life. Med Care 27 (suppl):5217–5232

Robinson R (1993) Cost-Benefit Analysis. Brit Med J 307:924–926

Rosser R, Kind P (1978) A scale of valuations of states of illness. Is there a social consensus? Int J Epidemiol 7:347–358

Tan-Torres T (1990) Comparison of different methods of eliciting utilities for outcome states in leprosy. Report to TDR/WHO

Torrance GW (1986) Measurement of health state utilities for economic appraisal J Health Econ 5:1–30

Torrance GW, Thomas WH, Sackett D (1972) A utility maximisation model for evaluation of health care programmes. Health Services Res 7:118–133

Ware J, Sherbourne CD (1992) The MOS 36 item short form health survey. Med Care 30:473–483

Williams A (1984) Economics of coronary artery by-pass grafting. Brit Med J 291:326–329

Williams J, Wood-Dauphinee S (1989) Assessing quality of life: measures of utility. In: Quality of life and technology assessment. Monograph of the Council on Health Care Technology, National Academy Press, Washington DC

World Bank (1993) Investing in Health. World Development Report 1993. Oxford University Press

The PCASEE Model: An Approach to Subjective Well-Being

P. Bech

Introduction

There are many ways to measure the functional state of an individual, and the number of proposals for scales purported to measure quality of life is growing at a fast rate. This indicates that few of the existing measures in this area are satisfactory. One of the reasons for dissatisfaction with the majority of scales in this area is the disparity between dimensions selected to assess functioning and those selected to assess quality of life. The PCASEE model aims to overcome this difficulty by adding a quality of life/satisfaction measure to each of the dimensions of functioning. The latter have been selected so as to correspond in general terms to the axes of the DSM-III-R because of the wide use of that classification and familiarity among mental health professionals with the way of using DSM-III-R axes. The PCASEE method addresses six dimensions: P, physical indicators; C, cognitive indicators; A, affective indicators; S, social indicators; E, economic-social stressors; E, ego functions. The model has been described in detail elsewhere (Bech 1993). These dimensions correspond to those implied by DSM-III-R axes (American Psychiatric Association 1987). Thus, P corresponds to DSM-III-R axis 3 (somatic syndromes), C to DSM-III axis 1 (organic mental syndromes), A to DSM-III-R axis 1 (mental (mood) syndromes), S to DSM-III-R axis 5 (social functioning), E, to DSM-III-R axis 4 (psychosocial stressors), and E to DSM-III-R axis 2 (personability disorders) (see Table 1).

Maslow's hierarchy of human needs (Maslow 1954) can be used to illustrate the level of measurement implicit in the PCASEE model. Table 2 shows possible areas of correspondence between the DSM-III axes of disability (ranked in accordance with the Maslow structure of needs), the objective Maslow needs, and the subjective PCASEE indicators.

McCall (1976) argues that the state of needing something is not a psychological state but a physical state and, consequently, an objective measure. In contrast, the question of whether a desire is satisfied is settled by asking the person about his or her inner experience, i.e., a psychological state. This illustrates the complexity of the relationship between objective and subjective indicators as used in this area.

The content validity of scales of subjective perceptions of health can be examined with reference to the PCASEE model. For example, scales such as the General Health Questionnaire (Goldberg 1972) and the Psychological General

J. Orley, W. Kuyken (Eds.)
Quality of Life Assessment:
International Perspectives

Table 1. The association between the descriptive levels of observation (diagnostic symptoms, ailment-oriented symptoms, and subjective well-being or quality of life) and the PCASEE repertoire (in brackets, the corresponding DSM-III-R axes)

Descriptive levels	P = Physical (axis 3)	C = Cognitive (axis 1)	A = Affective (axis 1)	S = Social (axis 5)	E = Economic stressors (axis 4)	E = Ego functions (axis 2)
Diagnoses or syndromes	Somatic disorders	Organic brain disorders of schizophrenia	Affective disorders	Activity of daily life	Psychosocial stressors	Personality disorders
Ailment-orientated symptoms	Tiredness, sleep, appetite	Concentration, memory	Melancholia, anxiety, phobia	Group-directed behavior, time structure	Stress behavior	Self-identity, self-acceptance
Subjective quality of life	Good health	Decision-making good	Good emotional contact, interests	Doing things well	Feeling economic basis good	Playing useful part in things

Table 2. The DSM-III-R axes and the PCASEE components rank-ordered in accordance with Maslow's hierarchical needs

DSM-III-R axes of disability	Objective quality of life components (Maslow's hierarchical needs)	Subjective quality of life components (PCASEE model)
Somatic disorders (axis 3)	Physiological needs (the lower levels)	Physical indicators
Psychosocial stressors (axis 4)	Safety needs	Economic-social indicators
Social functioning (axis 5)	Belongingness needs	Social indicators
Personality disorders (axis 2)	Self-esteem needs	Ego indicators
Mental disorders (axis 1)	Self-actualization needs (the higher levels)	Cognitive and emotional indicators

Well-Being Schedule (Dupuy 1984), are developed without a strict correspondence to the PCASEE model, but both can be related successfully to the PCASEE model (Bech 1993). These items reflect Maslow's concept of self-actualization to a certain degree.

Traditional self-rating scales like the General Health Questionnaire have been criticized by Thunedborg et al. (1993): "Their use implies that quality of life (*sic*) means the same to everybody and so can be defined in general terms. Even if the items they contain have been selected by studying an appropriate group of patients, the instrument may only strictly be applicable to a non-existent average individual." As a reaction against such group-oriented scales Thunedborg et al. (1993) developed a repertory grid for the measurement of individual quality of life. The PCASEE model was used to evaluate how the patient was before treatment and post-treatment, and how he or she wished to be. Using the same idiographic approach Stoker et al. (1993) developed another repertory grid method. Based on the latter findings Bech (1993) developed a questionnaire covering the PCASEE repertoire.

Treatment Efficacy Within the PCASEE Model

As discussed by Bech (1990), the concept of improvement during treatment should not only focus on the clinical distance between the current state compared to the patient's pretreatment position but should also take the intended goal of treatment into account. Hence, the patient's subjective assessment of whether the aim of treatment is satisfied becomes central.

The concept of improvement during a treatment trial is traditionally considered as the treating doctor's global impression of the change in the patient's condition when the current state is compared to the pretreatment position. The official instructions to the doctor for the clinical assessment of improvement are: Compared to the patient's condition before treatment, how much has he or she changed today? (0 = unchanged or worse; 1 = minimally or doubtfully improved; 2 = mildly improved; 3 = moderately to markedly improved; 4 = greatly improved to excellent (Bech 1993).

As discussed elsewhere (Bech 1990), the doctor's global impression of improvement of illness is based on an intuitive weighting of different symptoms of illness. The frame of reference is implicitly the symptoms of illness on which the treatment is supposed to work (Bech 1993) and not necessarily the general disability.

Health-related quality of life scales have mostly been used as outcome measures in clinical trials, i.e., as improvement scales. In patients with generalized anxiety disorders Thunedborg et al. (1993) showed that the repertory grid method had a better discrimination validity (sensitivity to improvement) than global scales of improvement of illness, disability scales or other health status scales. In the study by Croog et al. (1986) comparing different antihypertensive drugs, the Psychological General Well-Being Schedule was found to be most sensitive in measuring improvement.

Table 3 shows the most common side-effects of psychoactive drugs using the WHO Adverse Reaction Terminology (WHO 1990). The dose-related, pharmacological side-effects of treatment are common but usually not serious compared to the idiosyncratic, allergic side-effects of drugs. However, it is often difficult to detect the pharmacological side-effects because they frequently

Table 3. Adverse drug effects and quality of life

Quality of life components (PCASEE)	Side-effects of treatment (WHO codes)
Physiological needs	Insomnia (0183)
	Sexual dysfunction (0182)
	Weight gain (0408)
Other physical indicators	Headache (0409)
Other neurological indicators	Tremor (0154)
Other autonomic indicators	Mouth dry (0218)
	Nausea (0308)
Cognitive indicators	Concentration impaired (1127)
	Confusion (0092)
	Somnolence (0197)
Affective indicators	Apathy (0167)
	Nervousness (0188)
Social indicators	Fatigue (0724)
Ego indicators	Dependence (0174)

have different manifestations in different patients, and no single patient will experience all the potential side-effects (Table 3; Bech 1993). In this situation, quality of life measures important indicators of side-effects.

In this vein of thought, the United States Food and Drug Administration (FDA 1980) defines drug reactions as any experience associated with the use of a drug, whether or not considered drug-related by the treating doctor. When explaining an adverse reaction during a drug trial it is important to take non-biological factors into consideration, e.g., acute life events (e.g., DSM-III-R axis 4 or Holmes and Rahe's Social Readjustment Rating Scale; Bech 1993).

The global clinical improvement scale is most relevant in the acute therapy setting (short-term trial; Bech 1993). Compared to other global clinical impression scales the improvement assessment is most sensitive when differentiating between active drugs and placebo (Beneke and Rasmus 1992). Subjective quality of life scales should be considered as the patient's global improvement scale. However, as emphasized by Beneke and Rasmus (1992), a single global index score of improvement does not give any information of the content of improvement. This problem is solved using a scale covering the PCASEE model.

Conclusion

Health-related quality of life can be usefully measured in relation to the PCASEE model (Bech 1993). The PCASEE model provides a comprehensive assessment of a person's subjective perception of his/her well-being. This assessment can be related to other measures and classification schemes, such as the DSM-III-R. The PCASEE model has been used to measure clinical improvement during treatment. The first use has demonstrated the value of the model, which is being further tested in several ongoing studies.

References

American Psychiatric Association (1980) Diagnostic and statistical manual of mental disorders (DSM-III). American Psychiatric Association, Washington, DC

Bech P (1990) Measurement of psychological distress and well-being. Psychotherapy Psychosomatic 54:77–89

Bech P (1993) Rating scales for psychopathology, health status, and quality of life. A compendium with correspondence to DSM-III-R and the WHO systems. Springer, Berlin

Beneke M, Rasmus N (1992) Clinical global impression (ECDEU): Some critical comments. Pharmacopsychiatry 25:171–176

Croog SH, Levine S, Testa M (1986) The effects of antihypertensive therapy on the quality of life. New Engl Med 314:1657–1664

Dupuy HJ (1984) The Psychological General Well-Being (PGWB) Index. In: Wenger NK, Mattson ME, Furberg CD, Elison J (eds) Assessment of quality of life in clinical trials of cardiovascular therapies. Le Jacq Publishing, New York, pp 184–188

Food and Drug Administration (FDA) (1980). Procedural manual for handling drug experience reports. Glossy paper flow and algorithms. Department of Health and Human Services, Rockville

Goldberg D (1972) The detection of psychiatric illness by questionnaires. Oxford University Press, Oxford

Maslow AH (1954) Motivation and personality. Harper, New York

McCall S (1976) Human needs and the quality of life. In: King-Farlow J, Shea WR (eds) Values and the quality of life. Science History Publications, New York, pp 6–23

Stoker MG, Dunbar GC, Beaumont G (1992) The SmithKline Beecham quality of life scale. A validation and reliability study in patients with affective disorder. Quality Life Res 1:385–395

Thunedborg K, Allerup P, Bech P, Joyce CRB (1993) Development of the repertory grid for measurement of individual quality of life in clinical trials. Internat J Meth Psychiat Res 3:45–56

World Health Organization (1990). WHO Adverse Reaction Terminology. World Health Organization, Geneva

Quality of Life Assessment in Cancer

Quality of Life Assessment in Southwest Oncology Group Clinical Trials: Translating and Validating a Spanish Questionnaire

C.M. Moinpour

Summary

This paper describes the approach used by the Southwest Oncology Group (SWOG) to assess quality of life in cancer clinical trials. SWOG is a cooperative group in the United States that conducts clinical trials to evaluate new cancer treatments. Quality of life is assessed in selected trials, particularly those in which treatment aims are expected to differ minimally with respect to traditional endpoints and palliative objectives are of concern. SWOG's assessment approach is component-based and includes both generic and cancer-specific quality of life scales; the Medical Outcomes Study Short Form scales and the Symptom Distress Scale are the main standardized instruments included in the SWOG Quality of Life Questionnaire. Currently there is only an English version of SWOG's questionnaire. Hispanic Americans are the second largest minority group in the United States. Many Hispanics prefer interviews to be conducted in Spanish and many who can speak English do not necessarily prefer using English for reading or writing activities. Therefore, to avoid continuing to exclude Hispanic patients unable to complete questionnaires in English, we will be translating the SWOG Quality of Life Questionnaire into Spanish and conducting necessary validation research. A summary of the research plan is provided.

Introduction

The focus of this presentation is quality of life (QOL) assessment in cancer clinical trials as conducted by cooperative groups in the United States (US). Cooperative groups design and conduct studies to evaluate treatments for cancer with funding provided by the National Cancer Institute (NCI). Cooperative groups include hundreds of physicians, oncology nurses, and data managers around the US, usually associated with hospitals or cancer clinics/research centers. There are a number of cooperative groups: for example, the Southwest Oncology Group (SWOG), Eastern Oncology Group (ECOG), Cancer and Leukemia Group-B (CALG-B), National Surgical Adjuvant Breast and Bowel Project (NSABP), etc. Using SWOG as an example, between January 1992 and December 1992, 6249 registrations occurred on SWOG protocols, 59% of

J. Orley, W. Kuyken (Eds.)
Quality of Life Assessment:
International Perspectives

which were randomized comparative Phase III trials (SWOG 1993). This paper will address QOL assessment procedures adopted by SWOG, but the general approach is similar to that followed in other cooperative groups. Finally, a plan to translate SWOG's QOL Questionnaire into Spanish and to conduct the necessary validation research will be summarized.

In late 1988, a review of the QOL literature along with considerations of SWOG needs and constraints led to a decision to include QOL measures in selected SWOG trials and to the development of QOL assessment policies appropriate for a cooperative group context. Gaining approval for this new research from SWOG's Quality of Life Subcommittee and its parent committee, the Cancer Control Research Committee, and from SWOG's Board of Governors was important in increasing Group-wide support for QOL assessment in cancer clinical trials conducted by SWOG. A key figure in this process was Katherine Hayden, at the time a SWOG oncology nurse and chairperson of the Quality of Life Subcommittee. The QOL assessment policies were reviewed by researchers outside SWOG (e.g., Ivan Barofsky, Alice Kornblith, and Rosemary Yancik) and a summary was subsequently published in the Journal of the National Cancer Institute in 1989 (Moinpour et al. 1989).

Rationale for Collecting QOL Data

More patients are surviving cancer and are experiencing the tradeoff of *extended life* (due to advances in early diagnosis and treatment) *versus morbidity* associated with multiple diagnostic and therapeutic events and, in some cases, persistent, long-term side effects. Ideally, in addition to prolonging survival and disease-free intervals, treatment for cancer should reduce symptoms associated with the disease (e.g., pain associated with a tumor), not cause noxious side effects (e.g., chemotherapy-related nausea and vomiting), and improve a person's ability to return to a more normal lifestyle. Byrne (1992) noted that these goals are rarely met; particularly with advanced-stage disease patients, both the disease and its treatment degrade the well-being of the cancer patient. Granted, the usual endpoints in cancer clinical trials have been, and still are, survival time, disease-free survival time, tumor response rates, response duration, and toxicities associated with the treatment. Although alluding to the importance of the traditional indicators of cancer treatment effectiveness, Barofsky and Sugarbaker (1990) suggested that QOL assessment should be a critical modulating influence in their interpretation. In trials where cure is unlikely and palliation is the objective (e.g., protocols that address advanced or metastatic disease), QOL becomes the key endpoint of interest (Byrne 1992). Minimizing the compromise of patient QOL associated with cancer is one way to control morbidity until preventive measures can be found. In addition, by identifying survivor rehabilitation needs, treatments can be modified in ways to improve patient QOL.

QOL Assessment in SWOG Clinical Trials

Definitions of QOL for Cancer Clinical Trials Research

World Health Organization (WHO) Definition of Health

WHO's (1958) definition of health is multidimensional, addressing both the absence of morbidity and three aspects of well-being (physical, mental and social). Cancer patients experiencing pain identified the same three as salient (Padilla et al. 1990). Finally, WHO's current QOL project is broadening the scope of QOL assessment so that it is appropriate for research in a number of different cultures. SWOG's definition of QOL is based on the earlier WHO definition. Selection of QOL components and methods for assessing these components in SWOG trials has been largely influenced by the work of Ware and his colleagues (Stewart et al. 1988, 1989; Stewart and Ware 1992; Ware and Sherbourne 1992) and Aaronson and his colleagues at the European Organization for Research and Treatment of Cancer (EORTC; Aaronson et al. 1988, 1991, 1993).

Definitional Constraints

Excluded from SWOG's clinical trials-oriented definition of QOL are areas such as satisfaction with occupation, housing, etc., addressed in earlier QOL research (Andrews and Withey 1976; Campbell et al. 1976). This meeting continues the recent efforts of WHO's QOL project to broaden the scope of QOL assessment by incorporating domains and facets of QOL that are meaningful for broader evaluation contexts (e.g., freedom, personal safety, and security) and are relevant to setting social policy. Another objective of the meeting is to decide whether or not the WHOQOL should be further broadened because it might not sufficiently or appropriately address the QOL of special groups of respondents (e.g., cancer patients). In cancer treatment trials, although the special needs of different types of cancer patients receiving different types of treatment are addressed, broader dimensions such as housing or personal security are excluded because, in general, medical interventions such as cancer treatment are not intended to change these indicators. In SWOG trials, we find the term health-related QOL (Kaplan and Anderson 1988; Patrick and Deyo 1989; Patrick and Erickson 1988) useful. Broadening the scope of QOL assessment may make sense in cancer clinical trials when the research addresses long-term survivorship issues.

Patient Versus Proxy Report of QOL

In SWOG trials, patient measures do not substitute for physician measures but supplement them. With respect to QOL, however, patient report is viewed as more important because of the documented lack of agreement between proxy and patient reports. Sprangers and Aaronson (1992) recently published a comprehensive review of the degree of concordance between patient and proxy ratings, concluding that agreement is not very good and that additional research is required to identify conditions and circumstances that enhance agreement. Agreement is better when the ratings address observable, concrete aspects of QOL (Sprangers and Aaronson 1992). In general, 1) proxies underestimate the QOL of patients and 2) physicians underestimate the level of patient pain (Sprangers and Aaronson 1992). In large part, the discrepancy between patient and proxy report is the result of information that only the patient can provide. Although patient and proxy measures do not demonstrate good concordance, proxy measures can prove useful for patient groups who may experience cognitive deficits and difficulty continuing to complete QOL measures over time (e.g., patients with brain metastases).

SWOG QOL Questionnaire

This paper will describe components of the SWOG QOL Questionnaire. SWOG's selection of a QOL instrument followed certain guidelines: use of a categorical versus a visual analogue scale format; use of a set of core items that are generic in nature and can be included in any trial; use of a set of treatment-/disease-specific items that are to be revised for each new study; and use of scales with adequate psychometric properties. The generic items are provided by the MOS SF scales (Stewart et al. 1988, 1989; Stewart and Ware 1992; Ware and Sherbourne 1992) while the disease- and treatment-specific items come from the Symptom Distress Scale (McCorkle 1987; McCorkle and Benoliel 1983; McCorkle et al. 1989) and new items that are designed for each study. The Symptom Distress Scale is considered part of the core set of items because these items describe general symptom status for patients undergoing treatment for cancer regardless of the disease site or the type of treatment employed. Since the Symptom Distress Scale items are not totally comprehensive for this purpose, we have found it necessary to add items depending on the nature of the protocol. SWOG's experience assessing QOL of cancer patients would suggest that the WHOQOL may well need to incorporate additional items for special groups of respondents (e.g., cancer patients, patients with different chronic diseases, refugees). Table 1 summarizes the QOL dimensions assessed by the SWOG Questionnaire and the specific scales addressing each dimension.

Data in Table 2 document that generic scales such as the MOS-SF are reliable for cancer patients. Two of the three trials are ongoing studies, whereas the advanced colorectal study (SWOG-9045) just closed. Internal consistence reliability has yet to be estimated for the treatment-specific items.

Timing of QOL Assessments

In SWOG clinical trials, QOL is assessed at least three times: at randomization, during treatment, and at the conclusion of the protocol-delivered treat-

Table 1. Southwest Oncology Group Quality of Life Questionnaire[a]

	Instrument	No. Items
Primary Endpoints		
Disease/treatment-specific symptoms	a. Developed for Protocol	Varies
	b. Symptom Distress Scale (McCorkle 1987; McCorkle and Benoliel 1983; McCorkle et al. 1989)	11[b]
Physical functioning	MOS SF-36 Physical Functioning Scale (Stewart et al. 1988, 1989; Stewart and Ware 1992; Ware and Sherbourne 1992)	10
Emotional functioning	MOS SF-36 Mental Health Index (Stewart et al. 1988, 1989; Stewart and Ware 1992; Ware and Sherbourne 1992)	5
Secondary Endpoints		
General Symptoms	Symptom Distress Scale (McCorkle 1987; McCorkle and Benoliel 1983; McCorkle et al. 1989)	11[b]
Role functioning	MOS SF-20 Role Functioning Scale (Stewart et al. 1988, 1989; Stewart and Ware 1992)	2
Social functioning	MOS SF-36 Social Functioning Scale (Stewart and Ware 1992; Ware and Sherbourne 1992)	2
Global QOL	Uniscale from LASA[c] (Selby et al. 1984a, b)	1
Global health-related QOL	MOS SF-36 General Health Rating Item (Stewart et al. 1988, 1989; Stewart and Ware 1992; Ware and Sherbourne 1992)	1
Co-morbidity	Single Item	1

[a] Adapted with permission from Moinpour et al. (1995)
[b] The SWOG QOL Questionnaire uses 11 of the 13 Symptom Distress Scale items
[c] LASA, Linear Analogue Scale Assessment

Table 2. Quality of Life scales: coefficient alpha in Southwest Oncology Group trials. MOS Short Form Scales/Symptom Distress Scale

Trial	Physical functioning		Role functioning		Emotional functioning		Social functioning		Symptom Distress Scale	
	Alpha	n	Alpha	n	Alpha	n	Alpha	n	Alpha	n
SWOG-8994 Early stage prostate	0.90	92	0.93	95	0.84	94	0.76	94	0.86	86
SWOG-9039 Advanced prostate	0.94	417	0.92	421	0.78	426	0.72	423	0.84	412
SWOG-9045 Advanced colorectal	0.93	264	0.93	275	0.79	277	0.74	276	0.82	262

Adapted with permission from Moinpour et al. (1993)

ment. The number and timing of assessments are based on the natural course of disease, the treatment schedule, and the disease stage. Currently, QOL assessments are obtained at least four times during the trial; however, some Phase II studies have symptom assessment prior to each treatment course.

Proposed Spanish Translation and Validation Research

Demographics of US Hispanics

Hispanic Americans are the second largest minority group in the United States, accounting for 8.1% of the population in 1988 (Marin and Marin 1991), and represent the fastest growing minority group (Marin and Marin 1991; Ramirez et al. 1988; USDHHS 1985). The term Hispanic is a label, similar to that of Latino, and refers to individuals living in the US who were either born in or whose family comes from one of the Latin American countries or Spain. In the US, the three primary groups of Hispanics are Mexican Americans, Puerto Ricans (not living on the island of Puerto Rico), and Cuban Americans; individuals tracing family background to other Latin American countries or Spain are categorized as other Hispanics in research (Frank-Stromborg 1991; Marin and Marin 1991). Sixty-three percent of Hispanics are of Mexican descent, with 75% living in Texas or California (Westberg 1989).

Need for Spanish Translations

Marin and Marin (1991) reported that 25% of Hispanics speak no or very little English and that 63% speak Spanish at home. In the Hispanic Health and Nutrition Examination Survey (HHANES) survey, 38% of the Mexican Americans selected Spanish as the interview language (Trevino et al. 1991). Frank-Stromborg (1991; American Cancer Society 1985) reviewed the results of one survey indicating that Hispanics prefer information in Spanish. Walker et al. (1990) reported that, across different regions of the US, 51–84% of Hispanics preferred to use Spanish. Marin et al. (1989) found that 67% of participants in a telephone survey in the San Francisco area preferred Spanish for the interview language. Ramirez and McAlister (1988) summarized literature indicating that Mexican Americans prefer TV programs in Spanish rather than English. Although it is still the case that many second generation Hispanics may speak Spanish, they may not read or write Spanish (Walker et al. 1990). Therefore, Westberg (1989) has encouraged researchers and health care professionals to ask Hispanics which language they prefer to use.

Informal reports from SWOG investigators and data managers indicate that a number of patients registered to SWOG trials speak Spanish only or may speak English but are more comfortable reporting feelings/emotions and health status in Spanish. Because of the difficulty in translating complex psychosocial concepts, we do not allow on-the-spot translation of the SWOG QOL Questionnaire (Aaronson et al. 1991; Berkanovic 1980). A validated Spanish translation of the SWOG QOL Questionnaire allows Hispanic patients the option of completing questionnaires in either English or Spanish. Without a validated translation, we are forced to exclude Hispanic patients who cannot complete a questionnaire in English and cannot generalize QOL findings to this patient group. It is for these reasons that we are pursuing a Spanish translation of the SWOG QOL Questionnaire along with necessary validation research.

Spanish Translation Issues

Research has attested to the difficulty of achieving one-to-one correspondence in translating QOL, psychosocial, and health status concepts (Aaronson et al. 1991; Deyo 1984; Marin and Marin 1991). Berkanovic (1980) indicated the need for both forward (into the new language) and backward (into the original language) translations. Failure to provide a back translation of a health survey translated into Spanish resulted in a translated version with inferior psychometric properties. Berkanovic suggested that, by not checking the quality of idiomatic usage with a back translation, those participants interviewed in Spanish may have taken the survey less seriously. For this reason, our research will involve up to three separate Spanish and Back-to-English translations. Researchers who developed the scales will serve as consultants and review back translations of the questionnaires.

Variability in Spanish (both written and spoken) is considerable in the United States. We will emphasize the written Spanish used by Mexican Americans in the Southwestern region of the United States and in Southern California. The main translation should be appropriate for dialects spoken/read by Hispanics who are characterized as Mexican American, specifically in San Antonio, Texas. In keeping with the suggestions of Marin and Marin (1991) and Hendricson et al. (1989), the translation will target the dialect of this region of the United States. However, one of the questions of this application is the equivalence of a translation done in the Southwest for readers and speakers of Spanish living in Southern California. Where necessary, we will utilize synonyms to account for dialect differences. We may find it necessary to present questionnaire items in both Spanish and English, as did Hendricson et al. (1989). Our proposed translation approach is consistent with other suggestions made by Hendricson et al. (e.g., use teams of translators including a second bilingual person to produce the back translation, have external reviewers familiar with the target dialect review the translations, etc.).

Marin and Marin (1991) have cautioned researchers against translating questionnaires developed for non-Hispanic white participants and using the translated version with a new cultural group, in this case Hispanics. Even adhering to the best translation procedures can result in a questionnaire whose dimensions are not culturally universal. Marin and Marin (1991) advocate adding a final step in the translation process, that of "decentering" (pp 93–95) the questionnaire to reflect cultural differences present in the second culture. In this case, the original questionnaire would also be changed. This approach is consistent with the current WHOQOL project and certainly reflects the ideal design to follow. However, building a questionnaire from the ground up is not feasible at this point in time for SWOG because we have ongoing protocols using the single QOL questionnaire. However, we will evaluate the need to add items addressing any QOL issues considered important by respondents completing the questionnaires in Spanish. Focus group discussions among patients, patient comments after completing the questionnaires, and perceptions of bilingual data collectors can suggest items currently not included in the SWOG QOL Questionnaire that are culturally specific to Mexican American Hispanics.

Acculturation Issues in QOL Assessment

Acculturation refers to the changes in attitudes, values behaviors, etc., that occur when an immigrant group has contact with a new culture (Berry 1980; Marin and Marin 1991; Marin et al. 1987). Berry (1980) suggested that language use, cognitive style, personality, identity, attitudes, and stress change as a result of acculturation. It is therefore important to assess the degree to which acculturation affects the success (as measured by psychometric properties) of the Spanish translation.

A number of acculturation scales exist. The eight-item scale used in the HHANES (Delgado et al. 1990) was based on a longer 20-item acculturation scale developed by Cuellar et al. (1980) for Mexican Americans. Padilla (1980) and Deyo et al. (1985) have also developed acculturation scales for the Mexican American Hispanic subgroup. A 12-item scale that can be administered as a four-item measure was developed by Marin et al. (1987, 1991) and can be used with all Hispanic subgroups. The acculturation scale developed by Ramirez et al. (1986) emphasizes media and language preferences for use in public health education interventions. An example of one of the four items is "Spanish-language radio listened to" with response options of "all/some" versus "rarely/never." We will use the HHANES scale in our translation and validation project because it was designed for a Mexican origin population and received considerable field testing through the HHANES project.

Research Plan

I, along with co-Investigators Geraldine Padilla, PhD, Patricia Ganz, MD, and Gary Donaldson, PhD and a number of contributing investigators and consultants, have been funded to conduct a study through a special request for applications (RFA), Quality of Life Assessment in Special Populations; the RFA was sponsored by the Division of Cancer Prevention and Control (DCPC) of the National Cancer Institute (NCI) and the National Center for Nursing Research (NCNR; National Cancer Institute 1992). All participants, but particularly Drs. Padilla, Ganz, and Donaldson and our consultants Drs. Hays, Modiano, and Valdez, have contributed to the translation and validation design I will now describe.

Rationale for Selection of Patient Groups for Validation Research

We selected breast and prostate cancer for this translation and validation research because each represents such an important health problem. Current estimates indicate that one of nine women will develop breast cancer during her lifetime (Cancer Statistics Review 1983–1987; NIH 1990). Frank-Stromborg (1991) noted that breast cancer (along with colorectal cancer) is the most common cancer for Hispanic women. Other than skin cancer; prostate cancer is the most common male cancer (Boring et al. 1992) and is also the most common for Hispanic males (1991). These cancers also represent active sites for SWOG investigators and we would like to enhance Hispanic accrual on these (and other) SWOG protocols.

QOL Scales for Validation Study

Cancer Rehabilitation Evaluation System (CARES)

A short form of the CAncer Rehabilitation Evaluation System (CARES; Ganz et al. 1992), the CARES-SF, includes 59 of the total of 139 items (Schag et al. 1991). Psychometric properties of the CARES-SF have been documented (Schag et al. 1991). The CARES-SF is more feasible for use in clinical trials research and will be used in the validation phase of the proposed research. A total score and scores for the five main domains of the CARES are obtained for the CARES-SF. The CARES-SF was selected because it addresses a number of QOL dimensions and has been used with both breast and prostate cancer patients.

Functional Assessment in Cancer Therapy (FACT)

The second QOL scale selected for the validation phase of the research is the Functional Assessment of Cancer Therapy (FACT) developed by David Cella and his colleagues (Cella et al. 1992) for use in Eastern Oncology Group (ECOG) trials and other QOL research protocols. The FACT-G (v. 3) is the general or core version of the scale to be used with any type of oncology patient; it has 34 items. At the end of each set of items assessing a QOL dimension, a single item asks patients to rate how much that dimension affects his/her QOL. Reliability, validity, and sensitivity to change over time have been demonstrated for this QOL measure (Cella et al. 1992). Site-specific modules of items addressing additional concerns for patients have also been developed for the following cancer sites: breast (nine items); prostate (13 items); bladder

(12 items); head and neck (nine items); lung (nine items); colorectal (nine items).

Acculturation Scale

As indicated above, we selected the eight-item scale used in the HHANES (Delgado et al. 1990) acculturation measure.

Experimental Design

General Plan

The research incorporates three phases of activity: 1) translation of the SWOG QOL questionnaire; 2) validation of the translation; 3) a field test of the English and Spanish version of the SWOG QOL Questionnaire in ongoing SWOG trials.

Translation Phase

The first phase will involve three iterative Spanish translations of the SWOG QOL Questionnaire, including back translation into English and pilot studies/focus groups (Knafl and Howard 1984; Nyamathi and Shuler 1990; Stewart and Shandasani 1990) with small groups of prostate and breast cancer patients. The goal of the first phase is to obtain a Spanish translation (Mexican American dialect) that is appropriate for use in both the Southwestern region of the US and in the state of California. Preliminary Spanish translations of the two validation instruments, the CARES and the FACT, will be reviewed for dialect consistency with the final translation of the SWOG Questionnaire and will be refined accordingly. Focus group methodology will be used to evaluate the translations at each iteration. Of interest is documentation of the need for additional, culturally sensitive items for Hispanic cancer patients and whether or not both the Spanish and English items should be included in the Spanish versions of the questionnaire.

Validation Phase

The purpose of the validation study is to establish the equivalence of psychometric properties for the English and Spanish version of the SWOG QOL Questionnaire. Three Hispanic groups will be involved: Spanish monolinguals; bilinguals who prefer to complete questionnaires in Spanish; and bilinguals who can complete questionnaires in both English and Spanish. Non-Hispanic patients will complete questionnaires in English (i.e., patients similar to those currently completing the English questionnaire in SWOG trials). To address the issue of patient burden, we will administer a total of three QOL questionnaires to each patient; Hispanic patients will also complete the eight-item HHANES Acculturation Scale (Delgado et al. 1990). The three QOL questionnaires are the SWOG QOL Questionnaire, the FACT, and the CARES. Although most patients will complete all three QOL scales, bilingual cancer patients who read and write both Spanish and English will complete the SWOG QOL Questionnaire in English and Spanish. To keep the number of QOL questionnaires to three, these bilingual patients will complete either the FACT (prostate cancer patients) or the CARES (breast cancer patients).

Bilingual patients who are bilingual but prefer dealing with written materials in Spanish will complete the SWOG questionnaire and both the FACT and the CARES in Spanish. Hispanics monolingual with respect to Spanish will complete the SWOG Questionnaire, the FACT, and the CARES in Spanish. Non-Hispanic patients speaking only English will complete all three QOL questionnaires in English. A bilingual data manager will read the questionnaire to illiterate patients, whether Hispanic or non-Hispanic.

Field Study Phase

In phase three of the research, we will conduct a field test of the Spanish translation of the SWOG QOL Questionnaire in at least two SWOG clinical trials (Phase III breast and prostate cancer protocols). Bilingual patients will complete the questionnaire in their preferred language. Those who speak only Spanish will complete the questionnaire in Spanish. An acculturation scale will be completed by Hispanic patients as in phase two. Patients will also complete the SWOG QOL Questionnaire one month after study entry, providing a measure of sensitivity to change. At least 30 patients who speak only English will complete the questionnaire in English in each trial. The main objective of the field test is to evaluate the feasibility of administering Spanish translations of QOL questionnaires in multicenter, phase III clinical trials. However, we will also be able to compare sensitivity to change for both the English and Spanish versions. Because of the Group-wide interest in increasing the numbers of Hispanic cancer patients in SWOG trials and the quality control methods we have developed for QOL data collection, we expect to obtain a sufficient number of questionnaires completed in Spanish to compare psychometric properties of the English and Spanish translations in the multiple institution setting of clinical trials research.

Conclusions

We are heartened by the increasing physician support for QOL assessment in cancer clinical trials. Interest at the national level is also apparent. The NCI workshop on QOL assessment (Nayfield et al. 1992) allowed the cooperative groups to share experiences and suggest guidelines for assessment, quality control procedures, selection of protocols, and analysis. The recent RFA released by NCI/DCPC and NCNR documents Federal level support for QOL methodological research and is certainly welcome since it is extremely difficult for US cooperative groups to conduct validation research and other methodological studies without outside funding support. NCI's Cancer Treatment and Evaluation Program (CTEP) has recently outlined procedures for incorporating QOL outcome variables in cancer treatment trials (Gotay et al. 1992a, b). The Food and Drug Administration (FDA) is increasingly open to consideration of QOL outcome data in the licensing of new oncologic drugs, but its definition of QOL is less multidimensional and emphasizes a new agent's amelioration of disease-related symptoms (FDA/NCI 1990; Shoemaker et al. 1990). Several books addressing the QOL assessment have recently been published (Osoba 1991; Spilker 1990; Tchekmedyian and Cella 1991). New instruments are being developed such as the Functional Assessment of Cancer Therapy (FACT; Cella et al. 1992). Other questionnaires such as the EORTC QOL Questionnaire (Aaronson et al. 1988, 1991, 1993) are building a substantial data base through their use in cancer clinical trials. We applaud the WHO instrument development effort and could well use the resulting QOL scales in future SWOG trials.

Acknowledgment

Dr. Moinpour was supported by grants CA 61674, CA 378429, and CA 37429 from the National Cancer Institute, the National Institutes of Health, United States Public Health Service.

References

Aaronson NK, Bullinger M, Ahmedzai S (1988) A modular approach to quality of life assessment in cancer clinical trials. Recent Results Cancer Res 111:231–249

Aaronson NK, Ahmedzai S, Bullinger M, Crabeels D, Estape J, Filiberti A, Flechtner H, Frick U, Hurny C, Kaasa S, Klee M, Mastilica M, Osoba D, Pfausler B, Razavi D, Rofe PBC, Schraub S, Sullivan M, Takeda F (1991) for the EORTC Study Group on Quality of Life. The EORTC Core Quality-of-Life Questionnaire: Interim results of an international field study. In: Osoba D (ed) Effect of cancer on quality of life. Boca Raton, FL, CRC Press, Inc, pp 293–305

Aaronson NK, Ahmedzai S, Bergman B, Bullinger M, Cull A, Duez NJ, Filiberti A, Flechtner H, Fleishman SB, de Haes JCJM, Kaasa S, Klee M, Osoba D, Razavi D, Rofe PB, Schraub S, Sneeuw K, Sullivan M, Takeda F for the European Organization for Research and Treatment of Cancer Study Group on Quality of Life (1993) The European Organization for Research and Treatment of Cancer QLQ-C30: A quality of life instrument for use in international clinical trials in oncology. J Natl Cancer Inst 85:365–376

American Cancer Society. ACS Survey finds need for education program among Hispanic Americans (1985) Cancer Lett 11, 6

Andrews FM, Withey SB (eds) (1976) Social indicators of well-being. New York, Plenum Press

Barofsky I, Sugarbaker PH (1990) Cancer. In: Spilker B (ed) Quality of life assessment in clinical trials New York, Raven Press, pp 419–439

Berkanovic E (1980) The effect of inadequate language translation on Hispanic's responses to health surveys. Am J Public Health 70:1273–1281

Berry JW (1980) Acculturation as varieties of adaptation. In: Padilla AM (ed) Acculturation: Theory, models, and some new findings. Boulder, CO, Westview Press, pp 9–25
Boring CC, Squires TS, Tong T (1992) Cancer Statistics CA 42:19–38
Byrne M (1992) Cancer chemotherapy and quality of life. Cancer trials should include measures of patient's wellbeing. Brit Med J 304:1523–1524
Campbell A, Converse PE, Rodgers WL (eds) (1976) The quality of American life. New York, Sage
Cancer Statistics Review (1983–1987) National Cancer Institute Division of Cancer Prevention and Control Surveillance Program. In: Ries LAB, Hankey BF, Edwards BK (eds) NIH Publication No. 90–2789
Cella DF, Tulsky DS, Gray G, Sarafian B, Linn E, Bonomi A, Silberman M, Yellen SB, Winicour P, Brannon J, Eckberg K, Lloyd S, Purl S, Blendowski C, Goodman M, Barnicle M, Stewart I, McHale M, Bonomi P, Kaplan E, Taylor S, Thomas CR, Harris J (1992) The Functional Assessment of Cancer Therapy (FACT) Scale: Development and validation of the general measure. J Clin Oncol 11:570–579
Cuellar I, Harris LC, Jasso R (1980) An acculturation scale for Mexican American normal and clinical populations. Hispanic J Behav Sci 2:199–217
Delgado JL, Johnson CL, Roy I, Trevino FM (1990) I. Hispanic health and nutrition examination survey: Methodological considerations. Am J Publish Health 80 (Suppl):6–10
Deyo RA (1984) Pitfalls in measuring the health status of Mexican Americans: Comparative validity of the English and Spanish Sickness Impact Profile. Clin Res 32:293A
Deyo RA, Diehl AK, Hazuda H, Stern MP (1985) A simple language-based acculturation scale for Mexican Americans: Validaton and application to health care research. Am J Public Health 75:51–55
FDA/NCI Working Group on clinical trials endpoints agrees on broader approval criteria: Survival, response rates, time to failure, life quality (1990) Clin Cancer Lett 13:1–7
Frank-Stromborg M (1991) Changing demographics in the United States. Implications for health professionals. Cancer 67:1772–1778
Ganz PA, Schlag CAC, Lee JJ, Sim MS (1992) The CARES: A generic measure of health-related quality of life for patients with cancer. Quality Life Res 1:19–29
Gotay CC, Korn EL, McCabe MS, Moore TD, Cheson BD (1992a) Building quality of life assessment into cancer treatment studies. Oncology 6:25–28
Gotay CC, Korn EL, McCabe MS, Moore TD, Cheson BD (1992b) Quality of life assessment in cancer treatment protocols: Research issues in protocol development. J Natl Cancer Inst 84:575–579
Hendricson WD, Russell IJ, Prihoda TJ, Jacobson JM, Rogan A, Bishop GD (1989) An approach to developing a valid Spanish language translation of a health-status questionnaire. Med Care 27:959–966
Kaplan M, Anderson JP (1988) A general health policy model: Update and applications. Health Services Res, 23, 203–205
Knafl K, Howard M (1984) Interpreting and reporting qualitative research. Res Nurs Health 7:17–24
Marin G, Marin BV (1991) Research with Hispanic populations. Applied Social Research Methods Series. Volume 23. Newbury Park, CA, Sage Publications
Marin G, Perez-Stable EJ, Marin BV (1989) Cigarette smoking among San Francisco Hispanics: The role of acculturation and gender. Am J Pub Health 79:196–199
Marin G, Sabogal F, Marin BV, Otero-Sabogal R, Perez-Stable EJ (1987) Development of a short acculturation scale for Hispanics. Hispanic J Behav Sci 9:183–205
McCorkle R (1987) The measurement of symptom distress. Seminars Oncol Nursing 3:248–256
McCorkle R, Benoliel JQ (1983) Symptom distress, current concerns and mood disturbance after diagnosis of life-threatening disease. Social Sci Med 17:431–438
McCorkle R, Benoliel JQ, Donaldson G, Georgiadou F, Moinpour CM, Goodell B (1989) A randomized clinical trial of home nursing care for lung cancer patients. Cancer 64:1375–1382

Moinpour CM, Feigl P, Metch B, Hayden KA, Meyskens FL, Crowley J (1989) Quality of life end points in cancer clinical trials: review and recommendations. J Natl Cancer Inst 81:485–495

Moinpour CM, Savage M, Hayden KA, Sawyers J, Upchurch C (1993) Quality of life assessment in cancer clinical trials. In: Dimsdale JE, Baum A (eds) Quality of life in behavioral medicine research. Hillsdale NJ, Lawrence Erlbaum Associates, in press

National Cancer Institute, National Center for Nursing Research (1992). Quality of Life Assessment in Special Populations. RFA Number: CA/NR-92-27. In: Catalog of Federal Domestic Assistance No. 93.399, Cancer Control Research, and No. 93.361, Nursing Research, 1992

National Institutes of Health Consensus Conference Statement: Treatment of Early-stage Breast Cancer. (June 18–21, 1990) Bethesda, MD: National Institutes of Health

Nayfield SG, Ganz PA, Moinpour CM, Cella DF, Hailey BJ (1992) Report from a National Cancer Institute (USA) workshop on quality of life assessment in cancer clinical trials. Quality Life Res 1:203–210

Nyamathi A, Shuler P (1990) Focus group interview: A research technique for informed nursing practice. J Advanced Nurs 15:1281–1288

Osoba D (ed) (1991) Effect of cancer on quality of life. Boca Raton, FL, CRC Press, Inc.

Padilla AM (1980) The role of cultural awareness and ethnic loyalty in acculturation. In: Padilla AM (ed) Acculturation: Theory, models and some new findings. Boulder, CO. Westview Press, pp 47–84

Padilla GV, Ferrell B, Grant MM, Rhiner M (1990) Defining the content domain of quality of life for cancer patients with pain. Cancer Nursing 13:108–115

Patrick DL, Deyo RA (1989) Generic and disease-specific measures in assessing health status and quality of life. Med Care 27:S217–S232

Patrick DL, Erickson P (1988) What constitutes quality of life? Concepts and dimensions. Clin Nutrition 7:53–63

Ramirez AG, Cousins JH, Santos Y, Supik JD (1986) A media-based acculturation scale for Mexican Americans: application to public health education programs. Fam Community Health 9:63–71

Ramirez AG, MacKellar DA, Gallion K (1988) Reaching minority audiences: A major challenge in cancer reduction. Cancer Bull 40:334–343

Ramirez AG, McAlister AL (1988) Mass media campaign-A Su Salud. Preventive Med 17:608–621

Schag CAC, Ganz PA, Heinrich RL (1991) CAncer Rehabilitation Evaluation System-Short Form (CARES-SF): A cancer specific rehabilitation and quality of life instrument. Cancer 68:1406–1413

Selby PJ, Campbell JE, Chapman JA, Etazadi-Amoli J, Boyd NF (1984a) Measurement of the quality of life in patients with breast cancer. Rev Endocrine-Related Cancer 14 (Suppl):235–247

Selby PI, Chapman JAW, Etazadi-Amoli J, Dalley D, Boyd NF (1984b) The development of a method for assessing the quality of life of cancer patients. Brit J Cancer 50:13–22

Shoemaker D, Burke G, Dorr A, Temple R, Friedman MA (1990) A regulatory perspective. In: Spilker B (ed) Quality of life assessment in clinical trials. New York, Raven Press, pp 193–201

Southwest Oncology Group. Report of Studies (1993) Seattle, WA, Southwest Oncology Group Statistical Center, pp 5, 7

Spilker B (ed) (1990) Quality of life assessments in clinical trials. New York, Raven Press

Sprangers MAG, Aaronson NK (1992) The role of health care providers and significant others in evaluating the quality of life of patients with chronic disease: A review. J Clin Epidemiol 45:743–760

Stewart AL, Hays RD, Ware JE Jr (1988) The MDS Short-form General Health Survey. Reliability and validity in a patient population. Med Care 26:724–735

Stewart AL, Greenfield S, Hays RD, Wells K, Rogers WH, Berry DS, McGlynn EA, Ware JE Jr (1989) Functional status and well-being of patients with chronic conditions. Results from The Medical Outcomes Study. JAMA 262:907–913

Stewart DW, Shamdasani PN (1990) Focus Groups. Theory and Practice. Applied Social Research Methods Series. Vol. 20. Newbury Park, CA, Sage Publications
Stewart AL, Ware JE Jr (eds) (1992) Measuring functioning and well-being. The Medical Outcomes study approach. Durham and London, Duke University Press
Tchekmedyian NS, Cella DF (eds) (1991) Quality of life in oncology practice and research. Williston Park, NJ, Dominus Pub.
Trevino FM, Moyer E, Valdez RB, Stroup-Benham CA (1991) Health insurance coverage and utilization of health services by Mexican Americans, mainland Puerto Ricans, and Cuban Americans. JAMA 265:233–237
U.S. Department of Health and Human services. Health Resources Administration. Bureau of Health Professions. Division of Disadvantaged Assistance (1985). Health Status of minorities and low income groups. DHHS Publication No. (HRSA) HRS-P-DV85-1. Washington, D.C., U.S. Government Printing Office
Walker SN, Kerr MJ, Pender NJ, Sechrist KR (1990) A Spanish language version of the health-promoting lifestyle profile. Nursing Res 39:268–273
Ware JE Jr, Sherbourne CD (1992) The MOS 36-item Short-Form Health Survey (SF-36). I. Conceptual framework and item selection. Med Care 30:473–483
Westberg J (1989) Patient education for Hispanic Americans. Patient Educ Counseling 13:143–160
World Health Organization (1958) The first ten years of the World Health Organization. Geneva, World Health Organization, Annex *1*, (Constitution of the World Health Organization), p 459

Quality of Life Assessment in Cancer Patients in India: Cross-Cultural Issues

S. Saxena

The Background

India is a large, overpopulated, developing country. Its population is approximately 800 million. Of this population, about 70% is rural-based, 48% is illiterate and 30% is below the poverty line (DGHS 1991). A per capita income of approximately US$ 360 categorises India as a low income economy (World Bank 1993). Health care availability in India is grossly inadequate, with only 0.74 beds and per capita government expenditure on health only US$ 2 per thousand population (DGHS 1991). Sixteen per cent of the world's population lives in India, but health expenditure for this population is only 1% of the world's total. Disability-adjusted life years lost in India, 344 per thousand population, is the highest among all the regions of the world except Sub-Saharan Africa, indicating a high burden of disease (World Bank 1993).

The incidence of cancer in India is around 75 per 100000 (ICMR 1992), which is considerably lower than in the developed countries. However, the relatively low overall incidence rate seems to be a result of the pyramid-shaped demographic structure, with 39% of the population below five years of age. When age-adjusted incidence rates or age-truncated incidence rates are compared, India comes much nearer to most developed countries (ICMR 1992). It has been estimated that 0.64 million Indians develop cancer every year, which is about 8% of the world's total.

Inadequate awareness regarding early detection and scarce specialised treatment services result in a large proportion of patients presenting to health care settings at an advanced stage of cancer. Only a minority of patients can avail themselves of curative treatments because of the late stage of the disease and the heavy expenses involved. Palliative care is still not accepted by oncologists as an effective adjunct or alternative. The majority of patients are not offerred any palliative care. The concept of quality of life finds very little practical utility in the everyday work of professional caregivers dealing with cancer patients.

Importance and Relevance

The grossly inadequate public and private resources available for health care in India require a very careful assessment of cost effectiveness of all treatment

J. Orley, W. Kuyken (Eds.)
Quality of Life Assessment:
International Perspectives

strategies. In the area of cancer care, the traditional outcome measures, like period survival rates, have dominated medical research as well as practice. This situation has led to an undue emphasis on survival, hence on curative treatment. Quality of life has not been amenable to clear definition or easy assessment; hence it is ignored as an outcome measure. Measurement of quality of life is likely to result in a more realistic perception of utility of curative treatment and a more favourable balance between palliative and curative treatment. This is extremely relevant for India, as palliative treatment requires less capital costs, less technical expertise of personnel and is, overall, more cost effective. Assessment of quality of life is also likely to focus attention on the psychosocial aspects of cancer management, which will lead to better patient satisfaction.

India also provides attractive research potential, as quality of life assessment can be done on groups of patients receiving no medical services as well as on those receiving curative and palliative services alone or in various combinations. This complete spectrum of patients is likely to be useful in the construction of a quality of life instrument and also in subsequent comparative studies.

Cross-Cultural Issues

Quality of life cannot be viewed in isolation from culture. The WHOQOL Group has explicitly stated this in its definition of the quality of life ("...an enquiry into the perception of individuals of their own position in life in the context of the culture and value systems in which they live..."). Cultural beliefs about an ideal life affect the individual's perception of the quality of his or her life in the most fundamental manner. Hence knowledge of cultural concepts of an ideal quality of life is an essential prerequisite to the assessment of quality of life in a given culture. Cross-cultural assessment of quality of life in cancer patients promises to be a fertile area of research, as the influence of cultural factors can be studied on the relatively uniform biological substrate of the disease process. This paper discusses some issues regarding quality of life assessment in cancer patients in the context of Indian culture and its value system.

Concept of Quality of Life and Health

There does not seem to be an exact equivalent of quality of life in traditional Indian culture, but the concept of health itself is very close to what is currently referred to as quality of life. The ancient Indian science of medicine is known as Ayurveda, which means knowledge of life (ayu = life, veda = to know). Charaka Samhita, an ancient medical text believed to be written around 1000 BC, described two kinds of medicine, "...one kind is promotive of vigour in the healthy, the other destructive of disease in the ailing" (Charaka Samhita

1949). Together, these two kinds of medicine cover a wide range of human life, consisting of anatomical physiological, social, ethical and spiritual aspects for understanding disease and health (Balodhi 1987). The ideal quality of life has also been conceptualised as "sukham ayuh", a life which is not affected by bodily and mental diseases, is endowed with vigour, strength, energy, vitality, and activity and is full of all sorts of enjoyment and successes. A parallel concept is of "hit ayuh", life of a person who is always willing to do good things, never steals others' property, is truthful, self-controlled, self-restrained and works with careful consideration, does not transgress the moral injunctions, takes to virtues and enjoyment with equal zeal, honours revered persons, is charitable and does what is beneficial to this world and the other (Dasgupta 1952). The practice of medicine in Ayurveda involves understanding the individual's life and making appropriate changes in the way of living, rather than merely administering some pills and potions. The state of health and disease is explained on the basis of the interplay of the constituent elements of the body, the general and the elementary regimen and the influences of time and the season (Keswani 1974). Based on ancient thought, the state of health in India is conceived to be a broad and global concept represented by the following four interdependent dimensions.

Physical

Good physical health is indicated by capacity to perform vigourous as well as sustained physical activity and having a good appetite and adequate and refreshing sleep. Absence of pain and disability is also regarded as an indicator of physical health. Considerable emphasis is laid on diet, as different items of food are considered to have specific and profound effects on health and behaviour (Rao and Devi 1974).

Psychological

Psychological health is manifested by being in harmony and peace with oneself. The Bhagavad Gita (500 to 200 BC) describes a steady mind as a tranquil state in equilibrium, like "a lamp in a windless place which flickereth not" (Rao and Devi 1974). In the context of Yoga, one of the parameters of psychological health is conceptualised as the extent to which the mind is restrained from the constant bombardment of thoughts, emotions and sensory perceptions to attain a state of peace and tranquility (Varma 1979). Contentment with whatever one has is considered healthy. All desires and emotions should be kept under control. Emotions in Indian culture include not only anxiety and depression, but also love, passion, hate, jealousy, suspicion, anger, greed and many others. Excessive emotion of any kind is considered unhealthy. Habitual ways of thinking should be positive, but hopes and expectations should be in consonance with external reality. Behaviour should be guided by duties which have been specified for each phase of life.

Social

Social health is indicated by the individual being in harmony with others. Indian culture recommends interdependence rather than personal independence as the ideal. Dependence on others in the Indian context is a desirable state of existence and does not have the negative connotation which it carries in Western countries (Neki 1976; Varma 1985). Personal autonomy is not one of the ideals of human existence in Indian thought, in marked contrast to the Western way of thinking (Varma 1986). The individual in his multitudinous roles, depending on the phase of his life, is expected to fulfill all of his prescribed duties towards family and the community. Excessive attachment to nonliving things as well as living beings is considered a sign of ill health.

Spiritual

Awareness and understanding of the meaning of one's life, this universe and the Creator are indicative of spiritual health. An average Indian attaches much importance to spiritual aspects in daily living, and this does not seem to depend much on the individual's religious faith and practice. God represents an abstraction of the forces and laws of nature hence transcends the narrwo confines of religious belief. Spiritual aspects often attain even more importance when physical health is compromised.

The above four dimensions of health are recognised to be mutually interactive, so that deterioration in one dimension usually affects the other dimensions. However, Indian culture recognises and accepts that major disparities between different dimensions of health may coexist. A person with poor physical health may have good psychological and social health. Some patients suffering from advanced cancer report considerably enhanced subjective perception of spiritual achievements, simultaneous with deteriorating quality of physical health.

Unfortunately, in spite of the World Health Organisation's concept of health as a state of physical, psychological and social well being, practitioners of the "modern" system of medicine have largely confined themselves to assessment and treatment of physical illnesses. This fact is so well recognised by the patients and their family members that they have learned to report only physical symptoms to their doctors. A cancer patient rarely reports psychological or social problems to his treating oncologist, although these may be the most crucial factors affecting his quality of life. The contrast can be readily seen when the same patient seeks help from a traditional health practitioner or a faith healer, to whom he reports all the dimensions of his health and quality of life and receives culturally more meaningful advice. Many patients seek simultaneous help from hospitals and traditional health practitioners in an attempt to derive optimal benefit in disease control and improving the quality of life.

Assessment of quality of life can be made culturally relevant by aiming for a conceptual equivalence rather than a terminological equivalence. In the context of Indian culture, the quality of life concept perhaps needs to be aligned with the traditional concept of health to achieve this goal.

Quality of Life Within Family and Social Network

There is a strong sense of identity with one's primary filial group in India. Joint and extended families still exist in a substantial proportion of rural households. But even where the structure of the family has become nuclear, strong emotional and functional ties bind family members together. The quality of an individual's life is seen to be dependent on that of significant others within his family and social network. Deterioration in the quality of one person's life because of a serious illness like cancer seems to affect others in the family much more than in many other countries. In addition, quality of life questions often elicit responses which are relevant to the whole family, rather than the responding individual alone.

Quality of Life in the Dimension of Time

Quality of life is seen in India as a continuum along the dimension of time from birth to death. This concept of continuity of life goes even beyond the present life and finds expression in the belief of reincarnation (Varma 1986). The emphasis is more on how it has been and how it is likely to be in future than on how it is at present. This can be viewed as an inability or perhaps unwillingness to divide the longitudinal concept of quality of life into cross-sections. Hence, it is often difficult to make the individual focus on and report his present quality of life. Most quality of life instruments have a short reference time of a few weeks, as they are constructed to monitor effects of disease states and treatment modalities over relatively brief periods. This is likely to limit the applicability of currently available quality of life instruments in diverse cultures including India. In addition, cancer patients consist of subgroups ranging from acute patients undergoing active treatment, terminally ill patients and those in remission or cure with stable disabilities. These subgroups require different time frames regarding quality of life assessment. To obviate these difficulties, it may be desirable to keep the reference time flexible between a few weeks to a few years, depending upon the setting in which the instrument is being used.

Relative Importance of the Components

There will probably be marked differences in the importance assigned to the various components of quality of life among different cultures. One culture may place more importance on personal appearance while another does so on mobility. Even within the same culture, interesting rural-urban differences may be seen. It is imperative that importance ratings for each of the components be assessed in various cultures. This will not only lead to more appropriately weighted scores of the instrument but will also help in gaining additional insights into the cross-cultural concept of quality of life.

Besides the importance, even the polarity for some items may need close scrutiny in the cross-cultural context. The concept of dependence/independence can be taken as an example. As described earlier, Indian culture does not assign positive value to personal independence. This rather abstract concept surfaces in the behaviour and thinking of cancer patients, who expect and readily accept help from family and friends. Striving for independence by such patients is often considered maladaptive. These cross-cultural contradictions need to be taken into account when attempting to devise international instruments in this field.

Levels in Quality of Life

Indians seem to view the quality of their lives on different levels or planes. The following three levels are observed frequently in patients as well as in the non-patient population. The worldly, material level is the lowermost, in which the individual is concered with his health, physical safety, bodily comforts and material assets. At a higher social level, the individual assigns importance to family and social expectations, duties and responsibilities. At the highest spiritual level, the individual is concerned about the meaning and the reason for his existence, the universe and the Creator. At this level the individual ignores physical health, material assets and social achievements as transitory, hence unimportant. These levels are largely equivalent to the biological, social and existential needs of human beings described by Varma (1986) in a cross-cultural context.

During repeated assessments of quality of life, many patients may respond in a highly variable manner regarding the importance of an area, depending on which level they are operating in at the time of the assessment. The individual may shift between these levels in a complex way, either spontaneously or being facilitated by the interviewer. To a cancer patient, physical pain may be the most important determinant of his quality of life one day, but the same patient may respond at a spiritual plane the next day, dismissing pain as a minor and transitory discomfort and expressing satisfaction with his quality of life due to accumulated good deeds and a higher spiritual understanding. This phenomenon needs attention during assessment of quality of life.

Responses Tailored According to the Expectations of Others

Patients in India frequently tend to give responses according to the expectations of their family members and professional caregivers. They seem to be responding based on how they ought to be feeling rather than on how they are actually feeling. Often patients minimise their discomfort to please others.

Effect of Information About Cancer

A substantial proportion of patients undergo treatment for cancer without being aware of the nature or seriousness of their illness. Some of these patients may have a relatively better quality of life, as they may not suffer from the negative psychological and social impact of this stigmatising illness. On the other hand, deliberate withholding of information by informal and professional caregivers produces a negative effect on the quality of the patient's life. Assessment of cancer patients should include the level of the patient's awareness of his illness and the level of satisfaction with the information given to him as variables that affect his quality of life.

Effect of Trust and Faith in the Professional Caregivers

An average Indian patient reposes a high amount of trust and faith in his doctor. This may protect the patient from uncertainties and anxieties about his illness and treatment, leading to a better subjective perception of quality of life. The feeling of well being in Indian cancer patients does not seem to depend as much on the sense of personal control over the situation as is commonly observed in Western countries.

Cross-Cultural Methodological Issues in a Study on Assessment of Quality of Life in Acute Leukemia Patients in India

This section briefly summarises inferences drawn from a pilot study on assessment of quality of life in acute leukemia patients at the Institute Rotary Cancer Hospital, A.I.I.M.S. New-Delhi. While the results of this study are being presented elsewhere, the relevant cross-cultural methodological issues are discussed here briefly.

This was a hospital-based study on adult patients with a diagnosis of acute myeloid or lymphatic leukemia. Patients with acute leukemia were selected as the diagnostic group for this study because the quality of life of these patients is seriously impaired during the illness and treatment, but with adequate therapy the outcome, in terms of cure of the disease, is good. Thirty patients were studied during the induction phase of chemotherapy. The patient and at least one close family member were interviewed by a psychiatrist. The initial part of the interview consisted of open questions on the patient's and family's concept of quality of life and the patient's current quality of life. In the latter part of the interview three structured scales were used to assess the patient's current quality of life. These consisted of the Karnofsky Performance Scale (KPS; Karnofsky and Burchenal 1949), Functional Living Index-Cancer (FLIC; Schipper et al. 1984) and Beck Depression Inventory (BDI; Beck et al. 1961). Fifteen of these patients could be interviewed again in the early remission phase (4 to 6 weeks of haematological remission) using the same instruments. In addition, 10 new patients with the same diagnosis were studied in the late (more than one year) remission phase. The salient methodological issues brought out by this study were as follows.

1) The patients and their family members could understand and meaningfully describe many of the components of quality of life but they had difficulty integrating the components into the global concept of quality of life. This was partly because we could not find a suitable Hindi equivalent of this term.

2) The components of quality of life given most frequently by the patients and their family members pertained to physical ill health, negative emotions, forced confinement in the hospital, not being able to fulfill family and social responsibilities and financial difficulties caused by the illness.

3) The unstructured interview elicited considerable information on the effect of the illness on the quality of life of the patient and the family, but much of this information was not captured adequately by the instruments used in this study.

4) KPS was easy to apply and provided a useful global assessment, but its sensitivity appeared to be restricted to a relatively severe stage of the disease.

5) BDI was relevant and informative, but markedly restricted in its coverage as a quality of life measure.

6) Some problems were encountered in using the FLIC. A few items were perceived to be repetitive due to inadequate discrimination between the words used (e.g., feeling and appearing, hardship and disruption). Some other items were thought to be inapplicable for patients admitted in the hospital. Patients also felt that FLIC did not cover some of their important concerns, like financial difficulties and inability to carry out family and social responsibilities. The visual analog scale, although easier to use than point rating scales, still posed some difficulties for the illiterate patients.

7) The correlations between the scores of the three instruments were high (0.77 to 0.89) for induction as well as the early remission phases. This indicated that better performance, better functional status and absence from depression went together. For the late remission phase, the KPS score was a perfect 100 for all patients; BDI scores were low and FLIC scores were high. The correlation between the latter two was −0.46, indicating that in near-normal patients these two scores were not correlated as strongly as in patients with active disease.

Implications for Further Research

The conceptual and methodological issues discussed in this paper have implications for assessment of quality of life in cancer patients in India. The quality of life concept needs to be aligned with other related concepts (like the traditional concept of health in India) for generating culturally relevant items. Subjective perception of quality of life needs more emphasis than relatively objective measures. The reference period for the current rating of the quality of life needs to be flexible between a few weeks to a few years, depending on the need and feasibility. An effective method needs to be devised for assessing the importance assigned to each component of quality of life by the individual, over a period of time and integrating the information obtained, to derive a more stable index of importance. The polarity of some items needs scrutiny in Indian culture. Research also needs to focus on the impact of serious illnesses like cancer on the quality of life of other members of the family.

References

Balodhi JP (1987) Constituting the outlines of a philosophy of Ayurveda – mainly on mental health import. Indian J Psychiat 29:127–132

Beck AT, Ward CH, Mendelson M, Mock J, Erbaugh J (1961) An inventory for measuring depression. Arch Gen Psychiat 4:561–571

Charaka Samhita (1949) Shree Gulabkunverba Ayurvedic Society, Jamnagar, India

Dasgupta SN (1952) A history of Indian philosophy-2. Cambridge University Press, London

Directorate General of Health Services (1991) Health Information of India. Directorate General of Health Services, New Delhi

Indian Council of Medical Research (1992) National Cancer Registry Programme. Biennial Report. Indian Council of Medical Research, New-Delhi

Karnofsky D, Burchenal JH (1949) Clinical Evaluation of Chemotherapeutic Agents in Cancer. In: Macleod CM (ed) Evaluation of chemotherapeutic agents. Columbia University Press, New York

Keswani NH (1974) Medical Heritage of India. In: Keswani NH (ed) The science of medicine and physiological concepts in ancient and medieval India. Department of Physiology, A.I.I.M.S., New-Delhi, pp 3–52

Neki JS (1976) An examination of the cultural relativism of dependence as a dynamic of social and therapeutic relationship-I: sociodevelopmental. Br J Med Psychol 49:1–10

Rao AV, Devi SP (1974) Body and mind in the Bhagavad Gita. In: Keswani NH (ed) The science of medicine and physiological concepts in ancient and medieval India. Department of Physiology, A.I.I.M.S., New Delhi, pp 119–126

Schipper H, Clinch J, Memurry A, Levitt M (1984) Measuring the quality of life of cancer patients – the Functional Living Index – Cancer: development and validation. J Clin Oncol 2:472–483

Varma LP (1979) Yoga, meditation and mysticism. Indian J Psychiat 21:293–304

Varma VK (1985) The Indian mind and psychopathology. Integrative Psychiatry 3:290–296

Varma VK (1986) Cultural psychodynamics in health and illness. Indian J Psychiat 28:13–34

World Bank (1993) World Development Report – 1993, Investing in Health: World Development indicators. World Bank & Oxford University Press, New York

Measuring the Quality of Life in Breast Cancer

L. Fallowfield

Introduction

Breast cancer killed over 15500 women in the United Kingdom in 1992. Coping with the knowledge that one has a life-threatening disease and dealing with the side-effects of treatment exact a considerable emotional and physical toll. Although effective treatment means a reasonably good 10-year survival rate, the psychological, sexual and physical dysfunction caused by the diagnosis and treatments can produce a deleterious impact on the quality of women's lives. Unlike some of the other common cancers, there are a variety of possible treatments for breast cancer. These may have similar outcomes in terms of response and survival but may have profoundly different effects on emotional and general physical well-being. Thus, monitoring the quality of life in breast cancer is extremely important and can be useful in the following situations:

1) to assists both patient and doctor in decision-making about the most appropriate treatment option;
2) in clinical trials to help evaluate outcome of different treatments;
3) to identify women who might benefit from psychosocial interventions such as counselling or relaxation therapy;
4) to help inform economic evaluations and health-care policy decisions.

Different instruments to measure quality of life might be required, depending on the purpose of assessment. In this paper, the aspects of quality of life most compromised by breast cancer will be discussed, together with a brief critique of some of the frequently cited, but not necessarily most appropriate, measures that have been used in this area.

What is Quality of Life?

Definitions vary, but a consensus exists that quality of life is a multi-dimensional concept which includes specific core domains (shown in Fig. 1) including physical, psychological, social and occupational well-being. As cancer imposes threats to all of these core domains it is the disease state that has probably generated more quality of life research than any other. Much of this work has been in breast cancer.

J. Orley, W. Kuyken (Eds.)
Quality of Life Assessment:
International Perspectives

Core domains	*Typical items*
1. Psychological	Depression Anxiety Adjustment to illness
2. Social	Personal and sexual relationships Engagement in social and leisure activities
3. Occupational	Ability and desire to carry out paid employment Ability to cope with household duties
4. Physical	Pain Mobility Sleep Appetite and nausea Sexual functioning

Fig. 1. Quality of life

The Effect of Breast Cancer on Quality of Life

The psychosocial distress associated with the diagnosis and treatment of breast cancer has been well documented in both lay and medical literature. Early seminal work in the 1950s (Bard and Sutherland 1955; Renneker and Cutler 1952) described the primarily anecdotal evidence that anxiety and depression, together with impairments to physical and sexual functioning, were common sequelae of breast cancer. Later controlled studies (Maguire et al. 1978; Morris et al. 1977) compared the psychiatric morbidity of women treated for breast cancer by mastectomy with that found in women who had benign breast disease. These studies also reported considerable psychological distress amongst the women with malignancy. An intuitively plausible interpretation of these data was that amputation of the breast produced such a profoundly negative effect on feelings of femininity, self-esteem and body image that psychological and sexual dysfunction was an almost predictable outcome. This seemed especially true in Western cultures where breasts are symbolic of sexuality and femininity.

During the mid to late 1970s, there was a trend towards more breast conserving surgical techniques plus radiotherapy. This move was supported enthusiastically by many women and by those surgeons who had always disliked performing mastectomy. When randomised clinical trials comparing survival rates and relapse-free intervals in women treated by mastectomy or local excision showed no differences between the two treatments (Fisher et al. 1985), surgeons felt more confident about offering their patients a treatment which they felt should enhance the quality of women's lives, but not compromise their chances of survival.

As breast conserving procedures became widely available, researchers had an opportunity to compare the psychosocial impact of such treatments with mastectomy. During the 1980s and early 1990s at least 14 such studies were published (see Table 1). These studies have been comprehensively reviewed

Table 1. Psychological outcome of mastectomy (Mx) vs. breast conservation (BC)

Authors	Patients	Assessments used	Outcome
Sanger and Reznikoff (1981)	n = 40 Mx (20) BC (20)	Rorschach ink-blots Locke and Wallace Marital Adjustment (MAT) Secord Homonyms test and Body Cathexis Scale Minnesota Multiphase Personality Inventory (MMPI) Crowne-Marlow Social Desirability	No difference between groups in psychosocial morbidity Greater overall "body satisfaction" in BC group
Schain et al. (1983)	n = 38 Mx (20) BC (18)	Non-standard self-report questionnaire	No significant psychosocial differences, but less negative body image in breast conservation group
Steinberg et al. (1985)	n = 67 radical Mx (46) BC (21) (1/2 chose BC)	Profile of Mood States (POMS) Beck Depression Inventory SADS Non-standardised questionnaire on sexual functioning and social change	No significant differences between groups in psychosocial mobidity. BC group less self-conscious
Ashcroft et al. (1985)	n = 40 Mx (?) BC (?) (numbers unknown)	Leeds Depression Scale Spielberger Trait Anxiety Inventory (STAI) Locke and Wallace (MAT) Holmes and Rahe Life Events Schedule	Little difference between groups on psychosocial measures but better body satisfaction in BC group
Bartelink et al. (1985)	n = 172 Radical Mx (58) BC (114)	Non-standard 9-item self-report questionnaire	Less negative body image and fear of recurrence in BC group
de Haes et al. (1986)	n = 39 Mx (18) BC (21)	Cancer Patients' Symptom Checklist Non-standard tests of body image, marital satisfaction, fear of recurrence and death	Less negative body image in tumorectomy group No differences in sexual or psychological functioning or in fear of recurrence or death

Table 1 (continued)

Authors	Patients	Assessments used	Outcome
Fallowfield et al. (1986)	n = 101 Mx (53) BC (48)	Present State Examination (PSE) Rotterdam Symptom Checklist (RSCL)	No difference in psychiatric mobidity between groups, but more overt concern with fear of cancer recurrence among BC group
Lasry et al. (1987)	n = 123 Mx (43) BC + RXT (36) BC (44)	CES Depression Scale Non-standard body image index	Depression highest in BC patients who also had radiotherapy (RXT). Better body image in BC group. Fear of recurrence greatest among patients receiving chemotherapy
Wolberg et al. (1987)	n = 206 Mx (no choice) (96) Mx (choice) (56) BC (choice) (54)	Profile of Mood States (POMS) Health Locus of Control (HLOC) Locke-Wallace (MAT) Psychosocial Adjustment to Illness Scale (PAIS) Derogatis Sexual Functioning Inventory (DSFI) and other test	Psychosocial data (reported from maximum of only 39 patients in original sample) showed advantages to women who elected to have breast conservation in terms of anxiety and depression
Kemeny et al. (1988)	n = 52 Mx (27) Segmentectomy (25)	Non-standard questionnaire Brief Symptom Inventory (BSI) developed by authors	No significant differences between Mx and segmentectomy patients in "psychologic symptomatology." Body image benefit to segmentectomy patients
Morris and Royle (1988)	n = 30 Mx (no choice) (10) Mx (choice) (7) BC (choice) (13)	Hospital Anxiety and Depression Scale (HADS) RSCL	No difference in psychiatric morbidity between BC and Mx. Patients not offered choice of treatment more depressed and anxious
Meyer and Aspergren (1989)	n = 58 Radical Mx (30) BC (28)	Depression Scale from CPRS Adapted psychiatric questionnaire	No differences in psychological morbidity between groups. Less negative body image in BC group

Table 1 (continued)

Authors	Patients	Assessments used	Outcome
Maunsell et al. (1989)	n = 227 Mx (147) BC (80)	Psychiatric Symptom Inventory (PSI) Life events schedule Diagnostic Interview Schedule (DIS)	Significantly more psychological mobidity in BC group at 3 months. No differences at 18 months although psychological morbidity high (35%) in both
Fallowfield et al. (1990)	n = 269 Mx (no choice) (135) BC (no choice) (72) Mx (choice) (19) BC (choice) (43)	PSE HADS RSCL STAI	No difference at 12 months in psychiatric morbidity or sexual dysfunction between 2 groups; less morbidity in patients treated by surgeons who offered choice wherever possible

(Fallowfield 1990b). The reports emphasised different aspects of quality of life; for example, Maunsell et al. (1989) and Fallowfield et al. (1986) focused primarily on distress as manifest in clinical anxiety and depression. Others (Kemeny et al. 1988; Bartelink et al. 1985; de Haes et al. 1986) were more concerned with changes to daily life, notably effects on body image and/or sexuality. Because of these differences in focus and the extreme variations in methodology, sampling procedures and quality of life assessments used, the studies cannot be directly compared with each other. This is a problem bedevilling much of the early quality of life research. Numbers of subjects are usually small; thus the studies have low power and statistical analysis is difficult to interpret reliably, as studies with small samples require very big differences if statistical tests are to reveal any significant differences between groups. Futhermore, the newer statistical procedures of meta analysis cannot be employed. However, some general points can be made. Among those studies that have measured the effects of surgery on psychological morbidity, the consistent finding has been that levels of anxiety and depression are comparable, regardless of primary surgery. This surprising (and disappointing) finding – that breast conservation does not necessarily protect women from psychological distress, as had been assumed – shows the importance of broadening outcome measures in oncology to include quality of life parameters. Sometimes the effects of treatment are counterintuitive.

In general, whatever the primary surgical treatment for breast cancer, between a quarter and one third of women experience measurable psychiatric morbidity, which obviously diminishes the quality of their lives.

Body Image

Psychiatric morbidity is only one of the domains of quality of life relevant to breast cancer. Some studies have focused on body image and sexual fuctioning. A typical and erroneous assumption is that the primary focus of concern for newly diagnosed women is breast loss (see Fallowfield and Hall, 1991), for a review of this work). The supposition that body image concerns take precedence over many others, such as fear of cancer or recurrence, has been found in many papers based on rather thin data.

There is also a distinctly tautological element in work concentrating predominantly on body image. If a visible part of the body is amputated, it is not surprising that women report that body image is affected. However, mere perception of an altered body image tells us very little. Of more importance is the effect this has on quality of life. One woman may be dissatisfied with her body image, but able to function well in all other respects, whilst for another woman distress over altered body image may contribute to considerable psychosocial and sexual difficulties. This situation demonstrates the importance of looking at both aggregated and disaggregated scores from different domains in quality of life instruments.

Sexual Functioning

The WHO (1975) suggested that: "Sexual health is the integration of the somatic, emotional, intellectual and social aspects in ways that are positively enriching and that will enhance personality, communication and love." Unfortunately, the sexual well-being of people with cancer is a neglected area. Some clinicians feel that such matters must be of low priority to a patient with a life-threatening disease. Others may have difficulty discussing sexual matters with patients. Nevertheless, the loss of a sexual organ and of sexual function or fertility, together with the anxiety that a sexual partner might recoil from sexual activity, can have a devastating impact on the quality of life of an individual with cancer (Fallowfield 1992).

Few studies in breast cancer have explicitly assessed sexual functioning post-treatment. The findings of those that have done so are confusing. Many of the questions asked in some studies are ambiguous, failing to distinguish between the effect of surgery on body image and its effect on sexuality. They are not necessarily the same thing, as it is quite possible to feel dissatisfied with one's body but still feel interested in sex. Alternatively, one could have an intact body image but experience severe loss of libido. Assessment measures requiring a response to statements such as, "feel less physically attractive" (Kemeny et al. 1988) or "I feel self-conscious about being seen nude by my husband" (Bartelink et al. 1985), are not specific enough to determine sexual interest, as they contain both body image and sexuality elements. Often the distinction between what a woman feels for herself and how she feels her partner now responds towards her is blurred. Furthermore, few studies establish what the base line sexual interest or activity of women was prior to surgery, so that it is unclear whether lack of interest preceded or was a consequence of diagnosis and treatment. In two studies of women with breast cancer by Fallowfield et al. (1986, 1990) the level of sexual interest was measured via a self-report item from the Rotterdam Symptom Checklist (RSCL; de Haes et al. 1983). In both studies the sexual interest of previously sexually active women had declined in well over one quarter of all respondents, irrespective of surgical treatment. Another study by Kemeny et al. (1988) reported that significantly more women who had undergone mastectomy agreed with the statement, "Feel less sexually desirable now" than did those who had breast conserving surgery. However, there were *no differences* between treatment groups on the item "problems in sexual relations," with both groups reporting few problems.

Chemotherapy and radiotherapy can affect the quality of life as much as surgery. The impact of adjuvant therapy on sexuality was demonstrated by Penman et al. (1987). They found that women who had adjuvant radiotherapy and/or chemotherapy expressed more concern about physical affection, sexual relationships, and feelings of femininity or sexual attractiveness than women treated by mastectomy alone. Indeed, the mastectomy alone group showed no significant differences on any of these issues from women being treated for non-cancer problems. Likewise, Silberfarb et al. (1980) reported that radiotherapy and/or chemotherapy lessened sexual desire in women being treated for breast cancer. Some women also complain that they lose a considerable amount of sensation in the affected breast following radiotherapy or that their partners seem reluctant to touch the breast.

It is also interesting that many studies only monitor the sexual adjustment of married couples and fail to consider women who are living alone or cohabiting. As approximately 40% of women treated for breast cancer are not married, data on sexual activity derived from these studies are somewhat biased.

The relative impact that the diagnosis and different treatments for breast cancer has on sexuality remains uncertain, and more extensive research is required to enable analysis of correlations between treatment and relevant quality of life issues; such as psychological adjustment and body image.

Fear of Recurrence

Although survival is not compromised by breast conserving procedures, local recurrence is higher and concerns have been expressed that women would be more anxious about fear of recurrence following local excision. Some women are so fearful of recurrence that they develop obsessional checking of their breasts. Fallowfield et al. (1987) reported that 10% of their sample of women treated for breast cancer admitted to at least daily self-examination. Two studies (Kemeny et al. 1988; Bastelink et al. 1985) found that significantly more women who had had mastectomy reported fear of recurrence than those who had had breast conserving treatments. These results conflict with those found in another study (Fallowfield et al. 1986) which reported that breast conservation patients were significantly more anxious than mastectomy-treated patients that the cancer would return. Another group of researchers (de Haes et al. 1986; Lasry et al. 1987; Schain et al. 1983) found no differences at all in the amount of expressed fear between the two treatment groups.

One explanation for these differences may be that most studies used only a single item response from a questionnaire to determine fear of recurrence. It may be that data of this kind are too sensitive to elicit by such means and that in-depth interviewing is more appropriate. A study by Fallowfield et al. (1990) of 269 women reported that the majority gave "fear of cancer" as their worst thought, rather than "fear of breast loss," irrespective of the eventual surgical treatment received. Only 32 (12%) women, 18 of whom had a mastectomy and 14 who had lumpectomy, felt that losing a breast was a worse fear than that of having cancer.

Which Quality of Life Instrument?

Having looked at some of the threats to emotional and physical well-being provoked by breast cancer which impact negatively on quality of life, I will now look at some of the methods of measuring quality of life, commenting on how choice of instrument may be dependent on the purpose to which quality of life data will be put.

Measures Often Used in Breast Cancer

Commonly used measures, generic and either function- or cancer-specific, are listed in Table 2.

Table 2. Measures often used in breast cancer

Generic	General Health Questionnaire (GHQ) MOS SF-36 Medical Outcome Short-form (SF-36) Nottingham Health Profile (NHP) Psychological Adjustment of Illness Scale (PAIS)
Domain-specific	
a) Psychological Morbidity	Profile of Mood States (POMS) Hospital Anxiety and Depression Scale (HADS)
b) Physical Function	Activities of Daily Living (ADL) Karnofsky Performance Scale (KPS) WHO Performance Status
Cancer-specific	Functional Living Index-Cancer (FLIC) Cancer Rehabilitation Evaluation System (CARES) (previously CIPS) Rotterdam Symptom Checklist (RSCL) European Organisation for Research and Treatment of Cancer (EORTC) Quality of Life Questionnaire

Generic Measures

General Health Questionnaire (GHQ)

There are three different versions of the GHQ, containing 28, 30 or 60 items. The instrument was originally designed to screen populations for psychiatric and social morbidity. The GHQ-28 which has been used in many cancer studies, has four subscales, assessing depression, anxiety, social functioning and physical symptoms. Scoring is quick and simple and can be done using a Likert-type system or a bimodal response scale. The GHQ has good reliability and has been satisfactorily validated against clinical interview schedules. A threshold of five and more indicates possible psychological dysfunction. However, as the instrument was designed essentially for non-physically sick populations, it has been suggested that higher thresholds of 10–11 should be used for neurological in-patients (Goldberg 1986) or women with breast cancer undergoing cytotoxic chemotherapy (Hughson et al. 1988). The GHQ has been used successfully in clinical trial work with elderly breast cancer patients (Bates et al. 1991) and would be of value in screening those patients in need of counselling support. It has lower specificity and sensitivity than the more easily administered HADS and RSCL (Selby 1993).

MOS SF-36 Medical Outcome Short-form 36

This relatively brief but comprehensive and psychometrically sound questionnaire was developed for use for a variety of different purposes (Ware and Sherbourne 1992). It is an appropriate instrument in general population surveys for health policy evaluations as well as clinical practice or research in clinical trials. There are eight subscales in the questionnaire measuring 1) physical functioning, 2) impairment to role activities (due to health), 3) pain, 4) psychological well-being, 5) impairment to role activities (due to psychological problems), 6) social functioning, 7) energy and fatigue, and 8) general health perceptions. The SF-36 can be administered as a self-report questionnaire or by a trained interviewer. Currently an international team is conducting a four-year project to translate the questionnaire into 15 different languages (Aaronson et al. 1988). This group is also working on a utility index based on the SF-36 for use in cost utility and other economic evaluations. There are several different versions of the MOS quality of life measures, including a short-form 20 as well as 30, 36, 38 and 56 items versions. Of these, the SF-36 appears to be the most satisfactory, generic, health-related quality of life measure.

Nottingham Health Profile (NHP)

The NHP was developed originally as a survey tool (Hunt and McEwen 1980), but has been used increasingly to evaluate the outcome of medical interventions (Hunt et al. 1986). The authors of the NHP have conducted an enormous volume of research to refine their instrument and to produce evidence that it is both reliable and valid. The NHP is divided into two parts. Part 1 consists of 38 statements which can be subdivided under six problem areas: energy, pain, emotional reactions, sleep, social isolation and physical mobility. Part 2 has seven statements concerning the areas of daily life, hobbies and interests, and holidays. Respondents are required to answer 'Yes' or 'No' to statements such as "Things are getting me down." Each statement has a weighting attached to it, reflecting the perceived relative importance or severity of the item.

The NHP discriminates well between fit and physically sick people and it is sensitive enough to detect changes throughout the different trimesters of pregnancy. However, one of the difficulties with using it as a quality of life measure is that it only looks at negative aspects of health, making it impossible for patients to indicate well-being accurately. Zero scores do not necessarily reflect the absence of problems, and it might be difficult for the profile to detect relatively small but nevertheless significant areas of distress. This well-researched instrument has considerable popularity as a quality of life measure in view of its acceptability, cheapness and easy scoring. However, Sonja Hunt herself does not regard it as an appropriate tool for assessing the quality of life (Hunt, personal communication).

PAIS – Psychological Adjustment to Illness Scale

The PAIS is one of the most impressive comprehensive tests developed in recent years (Morrow et al. 1978). It was originally a semi-structured interview, administered by trained doctors, nurses, psychologists or social workers, but is now available in a self-report questionaire. The test has 45 questions looking at a patient's global adjustment to illness in seven important areas affecting quality of life: 1) health care orientation, 2) vocational environment, 3) domestic environment, 4) sexual relationships, 5) extended family relationships, 6) social environment, and 7) psychological distress.

The PAIS covers well all the core domains listed in Figure 1. The cost of this comprehensive coverage, however, is the complexity of scoring the test and the time that it takes patients to complete (approximately 30 min). Ratings for each question are made on a four-point scale. These scores are then converted to standardised T-scores found in tables in the handbook, providing a PAIS total score which can then be compared with published norms. The wealth of research done by the authors means that (unlike many other measures) there are norms available for a variety of patient populations such as cardiac, renal and cancer patients. The test has good reliability coefficients and correlates well with other tests measuring psychological dimensions.

Domain Specific Measures

a) Psychological Morbidity

The Profile of Mood States (POMS)

This questionnaire was originally developed in 1979 by Pollock et al. and later refined for marketing by McNair et al. (1981). It provides an assessment of an individual's current emotional state by asking subjects to rate how applicable 65 different mood descriptions are to them. Subjects are given semantic differentials, i.e., phrases such as "not at all" through to "extremely," which permit them to express the degree to which items such as "sad" apply. There are six different subscales on the POMS: tension, depression, anger, vigour, fatigue and confusion. Work has shown good specificity on the POMS subscales. It has been used in clinical trial work but is probably of more value in charting the benefits of psychosocial interventions. For example, Spiegel et al. (1981) showed that women in a professionally led self-help group with advanced breast cancer showed significant improvements over controls in negative feelings of anxiety, tension, fatigue and confusion.

The Hospital Anxiety and Depression Scale (HADS)

This scale was developed by Zigmond and Snaith (1983) specifically for use with physically sick populations. It has two subscales – anxiety and depression – and does not include items of a somatic nature, for example, tiredness, which could be caused by physical disease as much as mood disturbance. The test consists of 14 items, seven for each subscale, and patients rate items on a four-point scale. One further advantage of the HADS is that it is extremely easy and quick to administer, complete and score. (Few patients require more than two minutes to complete it and scoring takes about the same time.) Validation against the Clinical Interview Schedule shows that it has satisfactory sensitivity and specificity. Another useful aspect of the HADS concerns the fact that it has been translated into many different languages, including several European languages, Japanese and some Asian languages. This, together with the test's quickness, makes it a very suitable measure to use routinely amongst hospital patients, as it can be used with multi-ethnic populations.

b) Physical Function

ADL – Activities of Daily Living

The ADL (Katz et al. 1963) is a performance index which has stood the test of time, despite some reservations about its validity as a quality of life measure. Its primary use was in the assessment of the functional status of elderly patients in long-term care settings. Nurses or clinicians rate patients on six items: bathing, dressing, toileting, mobility, continence and feeding.

A major problem limiting the scale's usefulness in studies is its inability to discriminate well between differences in functioning at the upper end of the scale.

The scale has good validity and reliability and it has been helpful in measuring the functional status of, for example, elderly institutionalised patients. However, application of the scale in general population studies of quality of life or clinical trial works is not appropriate.

Karnofsky Performance Status (KPS)

The KPS (Karnofsky and Burchenal 1949) is a widely used scale of functional performance applied to oncology patients, and it does have some prognostic use, as pre-treatment scores tend to correlate well with survival. Despite its inadequacy as a quality of life measure, it is often used to make clinical judgements about a patient's quality of life and to influence decisions about whether or not certain treatments should be given. One of the many problems with physician-rated "quality of life" instruments that rely on physical functioning is the assumption that a patient with a lowish score due to immobility necessarily has a poorer quality of life than a patient with a higher score. A breast cancer patient, for example, who had recovered from her operation and finished adjuvant therapy would receive a fairly high score. However, she might be so emotionally crippled by depression and a concomitant loss of libido and self-esteem that her quality of life would be extremely poor.

WHO Performance Status

The WHO 5-point scale is physician rated; patients who are fully active and well score 0, whilst those completely disabled score 4. The same disadvantages already commented upon about the KPS are relevant to the WHO scale. This is an old instrument, unrelated to the WHOQOL.

Cancer Specific Measures

Functional Living Index-Cancer (FLIC)

Schipper and his colleagues have conducted a substantial amount of psychometric work on this instrument (Schipper et al. 1984). They have also performed concurrent validation studies against various measures of functional performance and activities of daily living, as well as standardised measures of depression, pain and anxiety. The authors of the FLIC eliminated any items that were contaminated by social desirability. The FLIC is a multidimensional instrument comprising 22 questions rated on a visual analogue scale, with specific questions designed to assess the overall functional quality of a cancer patient's day-to-day life, including items related to pain, stress, and the ability to work and do household chores. The phrases at each end of the scale represent polar responses to each question. Patients mark a line which is divided into seven equal intervals at the point that best represents their response. As with all visual analogue scales, scoring can be time consuming.

Some authors have suggested that, as there are so few items measuring each dimension of quality of life, its ability to measure significant change over time may be poor. Consequently, it is not recommended for clinical trial work (Maguire and Selby 1989).

Cancer Rehabilitation Evaluation System (CARES)

CARES (previously Cancer Inventory of Problem Situations – CIPS) is a standardised, comprehensive rehabilitation and quality of life questionnaire designed for use with cancer patients (Schag et al. 1990). It has been validated with other standardised measures of psychosocial distress, physical function, marital adjustment and quality of life. Patients rate problem statements on a five-point scale ranging from 0 "not at all," to 4 "applies very much," during the last month. The CARES contains 139 items, although not all items are rated by every patient, as certain subsections apply to some patients and not others. For example, the nine chemotherapy items are answered only by those patients who have been treated within the past month. The specificity of the instrument highlights those areas of psychosocial functioning of most concern to patients; thus its main value is to point out where interventions are necessary. Following each response box on the questionnaire, the patient is invited to indicate if this is a problem with which they would like some help.

Rotterdam Symptom Checklist (RSCL)

This instrument was introduced by de Haes et al. (1983) to measure the toxicity and impact that treatment for cancer was having on psychosocial functioning or quality of life. Respondents rate different items on a four-point scale by ticking a box opposite the reply which comes closest to how they have been feeling over the previous three days. There are approximately 30 items which can be divided into two primary subscales measuring physical and psychosocial dimensions. Additional items for assessment of treatment, or illness-related variables, are often included. Work is still in progress to establish population norms, but there are data emerging that show good sensitivity and specificity for the psychological items on the scale, and these have been validated against trained interviewer ratings. The test is extremely easy to understand and patients find it quite acceptable (Fallowfield et al. 1986). Furthermore, it is simple to administer and only takes five to ten minutes to complete. Scoring is straightforward and easy to compute. Hopefully the authors of the RSCL will be able to provide us with a handbook and norms so that the test can be incorporated into all clinical trial protocols and recommended for routine use by clinicians to assess quality of life. Some researchers add extra items to the core questionnaire that are relevant to the cancer site in question. For example, a breast cancer version has items relating to body image.

European Organisation for Research and Treatment of Cancer (EORTC) Quality of Life Questionnaire

The EORTC developed a multidimensional self-assessment questionnaire to assess quality of life in heterogeneous groups of cancer patients (Aaronson 1987). The EORTC questionnaire assesses functioning in physical, psychological and social domains, forming a "core" questionnaire. There are many studies being conducted to produce specific modules which contain other items addressing issues particularly relevant to different cancer sites, including breast. Hopefully, the meticulous care with which the authors are evaluating and refining their instrument (Aaronson et al. 1988) will prove to be a major breakthrough in the standardisation of assessment methods in cancer clinical trials.

How Quality of Life Information Can Help in Breast Cancer

Decision-Making

The primary surgical procedures for breast cancer in most Western countries are modified radical mastectomy or so-called breast conserving techniques, i.e., lumpectomy or wide local excision, followed by radiation therapy. Women may also be given adjuvant cytotoxic or hormonal therapy. As there is no difference in survival between surgical options (Fisher et al. 1985), women may be offered the choice between breast conservation and mastectomy. Good information about the general quality of life considerations can assist decision-making, and pre-treatment assessment of individual women can help health-care professionals in providing the best available support and advice. For example, Ward et al. (1989) conducted an exploratory study of factors influencing women's decisions about surgery. Of primary concern to women who opted for mastectomy was the desire to avoid radiotherapy, hence time off work and other side effects. Of prime importance to women who chose lumpectomy was the desire to maintain "body integrity." They seemed prepared to trade off the inconvenience of radiotherapy treatment for preservation of body image.

Clinical Trials

I have already shown the use of quality of life as an important outcome measure in clinical trials of surgery for breast cancer. They may also be useful in an adjuvant chemotherapy setting. In a study reported by Fraser et al. (1993) comparing different chemotherapeutic drugs and routes of administration in women with advanced breast cancer, no single factor pre-treatment predicted either response or survival more accurately than the patient's initial quality of life scores. Now that the case has been made for inclusion of quality of life in clinical trials as valid endpoints along with response, toxicity and survival, choice of test should be decided at the time that protocols are being designed. Quality of life assessment requires the same scientific rigour that is applied to other laboratory or clinical outcome measures. Consequently, it should be properly integrated into the protocol, not tacked on at the end, and adequate resources must be provided to permit accurate data collection and analysis. The "softness" of quality of life data is more often a function of the lackadaisical fashion in which it is collected or the manner in which tests are chosen, rather than problems with the measures themselves.

Screening

We know that up to a third of all women treated for breast cancer will experience significant psychiatric morbidity during the first two years of treatment, and that if these problems can be identified early, counselling intervention may help (Maguire et al. 1980). The problem is finding a reliable means of identifying those women most at risk of developing psychological difficulties. At least two studies have shown that it is possible to use standardised measures to identify factors pre-operatively in patients most at risk (Dean 1987; Maunsell et al. 1992). In particular, those patients with a clear history of depression and a high number of significantly stressful life events occurring prior to diagnosis are very likely to be strong indicators of the risk of development of high psychological distress.

Economic Analysis and Health Care Policy

Cost utility analysis (CUA) is becoming an increasingly important means of rationing/distributing scarce healthcare resources and QALYs form part of

CUA. Many criticisms have been made of the manner in which QALYs are generated (Carr-Hill 1991; Fallowfield 1990a). British QALYs tend to be calculated using the disability/distress matrix of Rosser and Kind (1978). More recently, attempts to operationalise the QALY can be found in the Euroquol (1990) and QALY toolkit (Gudex and Kind 1988).

It is important to recognise that as yet there has been little validation of the content of these instruments or of their reliability. Furthermore, QALYs take a macro look at health status valuations based on judgements of professionals or of those people who are generally disease free; they have very little to do with a sick individual's quality of life. The terms "quality of life" and "QALY" (quality adjusted life years) are confusing and this is more than just a question of semantics. There is a clear distinction between the sort of quality of life measures I use routinely in my work and those that tend to be used for the generation of QALYs. The problem is not simple and the issues need to be explored much more fully because the consequence of using quality of life estimates in resource allocation are scientifically and ethically complex. As a psychologist, I also have deep concerns about the notion that a judgement made at one point in time about the value of life in different disease states is a fixture upon which we can rely. My experience of working with patients, or with people who become patients who then either are in a state of chronic ill health or become cured, is that they show a great ability to adjust and cope with wide-ranging changes in their health state over time. Despite huge functional impairments resulting from disease, many people nevertheless maintain a good quality of life. If people in their well state are asked to make trade-off judgements, the data are of interest but do not relate to the judgements they would make in a changing or changed state when rendered sick by disease or treatment. Work looking at framing and labelling effects when eliciting preferences for different health states (preferences form the basis for many QALY valuations) shows that scenarios framed in the third person in which the word "cancer" appears convey negative connotations which influence any valuations made towards the lower end of a quality of life scale (Gerard et al. 1993).

Few can argue about the fact that we have finite health care resources but infinite needs, and some rationing system therefore takes place. Unfortunately, the measurement of quality of life, which can assist decision-making, provide valuable data in clinical trials, and identify women who need psychosocial interventions, has not been applied as successfully yet in economic evaluations.

References

Aaronson NK (1987) EORTC Protocol 15861: development of a core quality of life questionnaire for use in cancer clinical trials. Brussels: EORTC Data Center

Aaronson NK, Bullinger M, Ahmedzai S (1988) A modular approach to quality of life assessment in cancer clinical trials. Recent Results Cancer Res 111:231–249

Aaronson N, Acquadron C, Alonso J (1992) International Quality of life assessment (IQALA) project. Qual of Life Res 1:349–351

Ashcroft JJ, Leinster SJ, Slade PD (1985) Breast cancer – patient choice of treatment: preliminary communication. J Roy Soc Med 78:43–46

Bard M, Sutherland AM (1955) Psychological impact of cancer and its treatment. Cancer 8:656–672

Bartelink H, van Dam F, van Dongen J (1985) Psychological effects of breast conserving therapy in comparison with radical mastectomy. Int J Radiation Oncol Biol Phys 11:381–385

Bates T, Riley DL, Houghton J, Fallowfield LJ, Baum M (1991) Breast cancer in elderly women: a Cancer Research Campaign trials comparing treatment with tamoxifen and optimal surgery with tamoxifen alone. Brit J Surg 78:591–594

Carr-Hill R (1991) Current practice in obtaining the 'Q' in QALYs: A cautionary note. Brit Med J 303:699–701

Dean C (1987) Psychiatric morbidity following mastectomy: preoperative predictors and types of illness. J Psychosom Res 31:385–392

de Haes JCJM, Pruyn JFA, Knippenberg FCE (1983) Klachtenlijst voor krankerpatienten. Eerste ervaringen. Nederlands Tijdschrift Psychol 38:403–422

de Haes JCJM, van Oostrom MA, Welvaart K (1986) The effect of radical and conserving surgery on the quality of life of early breast cancer patients. Eur J Surg Oncol 12:337–342

Euroqol Group (1990) Euroqol – a new facility for the measurement of health-related quality of life. Health Policy 16:199–208

Fallowfield LJ (1990a) The quality of Life: The Missing Measurement in Health Care. Souvenir Press, London

Fallowfield LJ (1990b) Psychosocial adjustment after treatment for early breast cancer. Oncology 4(4):89–100

Fallowfield LJ (1992) The quality of life – body image and sexual function. Ca Topics 9(2):20–21

Fallowfield LJ, Baum M, Maguire GP (1986) Effects of breast conservation on psychological morbidity associated with diagnosis and treatment of early breast cancer. Brit Med J 293:1331–1334

Fallowfield LJ, Baum M, Maguire GP (1987) Addressing psychological needs of the conservatively treated breast cancer patient: discussion paper. J Roy Soc Med 80:696–700

Fallowfield LJ, Hall A, Maguire GP, Baum M (1990) Psychological outcomes of different treatment policies in women with early breast cancer outside a clinical trial. Brit Med J 301:575–580

Fallowfield LJ, Hall A (1991) Psychosocial and sexual impact of diagnosis and treatment of breast cancer. Brit Med Bull 48(2):388–399

Fisher B, Bauer M, Margolese R, Poisson R, Pilch Y, Redmond C, Fisher E, Wolmark N, Deutsch M, Montague E, Saffer E, Wickerham L, Lerner H, Glass A, Shibata H, Deckers P, Ketcham A, Oishi R, Russell I (1985) Five-year results of a randomised clinical trial comparing total mastectomy and segmental mastectomy with or without radiation in the treatment of breast cancer. New Engl J Med 312:665–673

Fraser SCA, Dobbs HJ, Ebbs SR, Fallowfield LJ, Bates H, Baum M (1993) Combination or mild single agent chemotherapy for advanced breast cancer? CMF vs. epirubicin measuring quality of life. Brit J Cancer 67:402–406

Gerard K, Dobson M, Hall J (1993) Framing and labelling effects in health descriptions: Quality adjusted life years for treatment of breast cancer. J Clin Epidemiol 46(1):77–84

Goldberg D (1986) Use of the General Health Questionnaire in clinical work. Brit Med J 293:1188–1189

Gudex C, Kind P (1988) The QALY toolkit. Discussion Paper No. 38. York Centre for Health Economics, Health Economics Consortium

Hughson AVM, Cooper AF, McArdle CS, Smith DC (1988) Validity of the General Health Questionnaire and its subscales in patients receiving chemotherapy for early breast cancer. J Psychosom Res 32(4/5):393–402

Hunt S, McEwen J (1980) The development of a subjective health indicator. Sociol Health Illness 2(3):231–246

Hunt S, McEwen J, McKenna S (1986) Measuring Health Status. London, Croom Helm
Karnofsky DA, Burchenal JH (1949) The clinical evaluation of chemotherapeutic agents in cancer. In: Mac Leod CM (ed) Evaluation of chemotherapeutic agents. Columbia University Press, New Yor, pp 191–205
Katz ST, Ford AB, Mosowitz RW, Jackson BA, Jaffe MW (1963) Studies of illness in the aged. JAMA 185:914.919
Kemeny MM, Wellisch DK, Schain WS (1988) Psychosocial outcome in a randomised surgical trial for treatment of primary breast cancer. Cancer 62:1231–1237
Lasry JCM, Margolese RG, Poisson R, Shibata H, Fleischer D, Lafleur D, Legault S, Taillefer S (1987) Depression and body image following mastectomy and lumpectomy. J Chron Dis 40:529–534
Maguire GP, Selby P (1989) Assessing quality of life in cancer patients. Brit J Cancer 60:437–440
Maguire GP, Lee EG, Bevington DJ, Kuchemann CS, Carbtree RJ, Cornell CE (1978) Psychiatric problems in the first year after mastectomy. Brit Med J 279:963–965
Maguire GP, Tait A, Brooke M, Thomas C, Sellwood R (1980) Effect of counselling on the psychiatric morbidity associated with mastectomy. Brit Med J 281:1454–1456
Maunsell E, Brisson J, Deschenes L (1989) Psychological distress after initial treatment for breast cancer: a comparison of partial and total mastectomy. J Clin Epidemiol 42:765–771
Maunsell E, Brisson J, Deschenes L (1992) Psychological distress after initial treatment for breast cancer. Cancer 70:120–125
McNair DM, Lorr M, Doppleman LF (1981) EITS manual for the Profile of Mood States. San Diego, Educational and Industrial Testing Service
Meyer L, Aspergren K (1989) Long term psychological sequelae of mastectomy and breast conserving treament for breast cancer. Acta Oncol 28:13–18
Morris J, Royle GJ (1988) Offering patients a choice of surgery for early breast cancer: a reduction in anxiety and depression in patients and their husbands. Soc Sci Med 26(6):583–585
Morris T, Greer S, White P (1977) Psychological and social adjustment to mastectomy. A 2-year follow-up study. Cancer 40:2381–2387
Morrow GR, Chiarello RJ, Derogatis LR (1978) A new scale for assessing patients' psychological adjustment to medical illness (PAIS). Psychol Med 8:605–610
Penman DT, Bloom JR, Fotopolous S (1987) The impact of mastectomy on self-concept and social function: a combined cross-sectional and longitudinal study with comparison groups. In: Stillman S (ed) Women and Cancer. New York, The Haworth Press Inc.
Pollock V, Cho DW, Reker D, Volavka J (1979) Profile of Mood States: the factors and their physiological correlates. J Nerv Ment Dis 167:612
Renneker R, Cutler M (1952) Psychological problems of adjustment to cancer of the breast. J Am Med Assoc 148:833–839
Rosser R, Kind P (1978) A scale for valuations of states of illness: Is there a consensus? Int J Epidemiol 7:347–357
Sanger CK, Reznikoff M (1981) A comparison of the psychological effects of breast-saving procedures with the modified radical mastectomy. Cancer 48:2341–2346
Schag CC, Heinrich RL, Aadland R, Ganz PA (1990) Assessing problems of cancer patients: Psychometric properties of the Cancer Inventory of Problem Situations. Health Psychol 9:83–102
Schain W, Edwards BK, Gorrell CR, de Moss EV, Lippman ME, Gerber LH, Lichter AS (1983) Psychosocial and physical outcomes of primary breast cancer therapy: mastectomy vs. excisional biopsy and irradiation. Brit Cancer Res Treat 3:377–382
Schipper H, Clinch J, McMurray A, Levitt M (1984) Measuring the quality of life of cancer patients: The functional living index – cancer: Development and validation. J Clin Oncol 2:472–483
Selby P (1993) Measuring the quality of life of patients with cancer. In: Walker SR, Rosser R (eds) Quality of life assessment: key issues in the 1990s. London, Kluwer Academic Publishers

Silberfarb PM, Maurer HL, Crouthamel CS (1980) Psychosocial aspects of neoplastic disease I: functional status of breast cancer patients during different treatment regimens. Am J Psychiat 137(4):450–455

Spiegel D, Bloom J, Yalom I (1981) Group support for patients with metastatic cancer: a randomised prospective outcome study. Arch of Gen Psychiat 38:527–537

Steinberg MD, Juliano MS, Wise L (1985) Psychological outcome of lumpectomy vs. mastectomy in the treatment of breast cancer. Am J Psychiat 143:34–39

Ward S, Heidrich S, Wolberg W (1989) Factors women take into account when deciding upon type of surgery for breast cancer. Ca Nurs 12(6):344–351

Ware JE, Sherbourne CD (1992) The MOS 36-item short-form health survey (SF-36). Med Care 30(6):473–483

Wolberg WH, Tanner MA, Romsaas EP (1987) Factors influencing options in primary breast cancer treatment. J Clin Oncol 5(1):68–74

World Health Organisation (1975) WHO Technical Reports Series 572:75, Geneva, Switzerland

Zigmond AS, Snaith RP (1983) The Hospital Anxiety and Depression Scale. Acta Psychiatr Scand 67:361–370

Quality of Life Assessment in Specific Populations

The Experiences and Quality of Life of Informal Caregivers

H. Herrman, H. Schofield, B. Murphy, and B. Singh

Summary

With increasing rates of disability and a major shift from custodial to community care, there is an increasing reliance on families and other supporters of people of all ages with severe and chronic mental or physical disabilities. At the same time there is growing evidence about the potentially negative impact of caregiving on the health and well-being of family caregivers. There is little systematic knowledge about the prevalence of caregiving and its impact on the caregiver. In past research on caregivers, study samples have been small, mostly recruited from service providers or support organizations, and hence unrepresentative. Research has tended to focus on a particular disability. The present study is population-based and cross-diagnostic, based on the assumption that other factors besides type of disability are influential in determining the impact of caregiving on the family caregiver.

As the first stage in an integrated research and health promotion programme for informal caregivers, a random survey of Victorian households is being conducted by telephone. The study aims to provide information on the prevalence of caregiving and to establish the broad spectrum of caregiving roles in the community without using predefined exclusion criteria, to assess the impact of the experience of caregiving on the quality of life of caregivers, and to identify services and strategies used by caregivers which help to minimise the negative impact of caregiving. Findings from the first wave of data collection in this survey are presented.

Use of self-identification as the method of recruiting participants resulted in the inclusion of a broad diversity of special needs caregivers. In spite of this diversity, covering a spectrum of caring roles, there are clear differences between this group and a comparison group of general caregivers in relation to health and well-being. The self-report measures employed in this work appear to be useful pointers to quality of life of the caregivers in our community.

Introduction

The quality of life of informal caregivers is becoming increasingly relevant to clinicians and to planners of health, welfare and housing services. Informal

J. Orley, W. Kuyken (Eds.)
Quality of Life Assessment:
International Perspectives

caregivers are members of the families and other supporters of people of all ages with severe and chronic mental or physical disabilities. With an ageing population, increasing rates of disability and the growth in "community care," the role of the family caregivers has expanded in recent years and will continue to expand. It is not surprising, therefore, that family or informal caregiving is becoming a major focus of interest for researchers and government policymakers (Lefley 1987; Levin et al. 1989; Zarit and Toseland 1989).

In many parts of the world there is a general view that, either for economic or humanitarian reasons, it is better for people to live in the community than in institutions when they have a mental or physical disorder. While this may be generally true, some families seek institutional care for a disabled relative or have institutional care urged upon them by health professionals. This situation suggests that there is a point at which home-based care or community-based care is not practical or desirable for either the caregiver, the person with the disability or the professional.

There are several possible reasons for arriving at this point. It may be that the physical or mental decline of the disabled person is such that he or she requires nursing or other care from professionals in an institution. Alternatively, the caregivers may have found that they are no longer able or willing to cope with the demands of the situation. What characterises those situations in which a caregiver feels unable to cope ("breaks down") or unwilling to continue ("rejects the care recipient") and seeks help or institutionalisation for a person with a disability is largely unexplored.

Investigations to date suggest that caregivers often experience hardship and may themselves suffer psychiatric disorders such as anxiety and depression (Braithwaite 1990; Fadden et al. 1987; Morris et al. 1988; Romans-Clarkson et al. 1986; Wasow 1985). Research in this area has been motivated largely by a concern for the mental health of caregivers. Caregivers are seen as "hidden patients." This motivation is not surprising and neither is the development of the notion of "the burden of care" as the general description of the research area.

However, the work in this area is limited in several ways. Sampling and methodological problems often mean that findings cannot be generalised beyond the study sample, which is frequently small. There is little information on the prevalence or types of the experience of caregiving in our communities or about the range of caregivers' responses or service needs. With some notable exceptions, there are few population-based studies (Green 1985; Stone et al. 1987). Much of the past work has focussed on families identified from contact with specialist services or with support organisations (Gwyther and George 1986; Fadden et al. 1987; Stone et al. 1987; Hooyman and Kiyak 1991).

The effect of this sampling bias in the literature is that we have little idea of the variety of responses to caregiving. The research perpetuates the notion that caregiving is wholly stressful and burdensome, by measurement with instruments which have been developed with the particular samples observed. This frame of reference limits the ways in which the experiences of caregivers, and their quality of life, may be conceptualised.

In addition, very little is known about the experience and well-being of caregivers relative to "non-caregivers" (that is, people not caring for others with special needs), or about changes for caregivers over a period of care. Neither do we have a clear view of the associations between personal and environmental factors and the effects of caregiving. It has been difficult to draw conclusions because of limitations in the studies – small sample sizes, cross-sectional study design, lack of comparison groups and unsatisfactory control of confounding factors (Baumgarten 1989) – although many interesting questions have been raised.

The experience of care will vary with the ages and other personal attributes of the caregivers and the disabled persons, with the social and physical circumstances of life, the duration of care, and with several aspects of the disability including its type, severity and stability. Several writers consider the likely process of adaptation to a severe and chronic disability in a relative as akin to the process of grieving after bereavement (Braithwaite 1992). Social policies and the availability of services are also likely to be relevant (MacCarthy et al. 1989a, b). The age of the disabled person and the type of illness are, in other words, only two of a number of factors likely to be important in determining a caregiver's response. Spouses caring for spouses and children caring for their parents are likely, for instance, to have very different experiences. Conversely, the middle-aged women caring for disabled children or young adults, and those caring for elderly parents, will have a number of things in common. Despite this, there are only a few examples of cross-diagnostic work (Draper et al. 1992; Wasow 1985; Whittick 1988). Measures to assess the impact of care have been developed separately, and apparently without detailed consideration of common areas of concern (see below). Analysis of the experience of caregiving has so far been split along disability lines (Fitting et al. 1986; Horowitz 1985; Jutras and Veilleux 1991; Harper and Lund 1990; Trute 1990; Sherman and Cocozza 1984).

Services for caregivers have been proposed and developed in many places and with various diagnoses. There is a rich experience, especially for relatives of frail elderly people (Braithwaite 1986; Schultz and Schultz 1990; Gallagher et al. 1989; Brodaty and Gresham 1989; Wells and Jorm 1987), parents of children with intellectual disabilities (Dupont 1986), and relatives of persons with chronic psychiatric disabilities (MacCarthy et al. 1989a, b; Smith and Birchwood 1987). However, studies of the elderly indicate that interventions, such as group support or education, respite care, or other domiciliary services, are not widely used, at least partly because the caregivers are unaware of the services available (Kinnear and Graycar 1984; Gibson 1984; O'Connor et al. 1988). It is likely that personal and social factors, other than the diagnosis of the care recipient, are relevant to the type of service found useful and acceptable. However, evaluative studies are rare, and there are few longitudinal studies (Zarit and Toseland 1989; Brodaty and Gresham 1989; Gallagher et al. 1989; Zarit 1989; Morris et al. 1988).

Overall, theory is lagging behind empirical work in this area and provides limited guidance to thinking about the important influences on the quality of life of caregivers. This is reflected in:

1) the lack of a common definition of "caregiving;"
2) the lack of an agreed theoretical basis for the assessment of the experience of caregiving and;
3) a limited theoretical basis for understanding the relationship between diverse factors and the experience and impact of caregiving.

We discuss these points here in relation to the design and early findings of a programme of research and health promotion for caregivers in Victoria, Australia.

The Carers' Programme

The Victorian Health Promotion Foundation is supporting a research and intervention programme focussing on the well-being of families caring for people with a range of severe and long-term illnesses and disabilities (Herman et al. 1993). The study aims to provide information on the prevalence of caregiving and to establish the broad spectrum of caregiving roles in the community without using predefined exclusion criteria, to assess the impact of the experience of caregiving on the psychological and physical well-being of caregivers, and to identify services and strategies used by caregivers which help to minimise the negative impact of caring.

The study is population-based, longitudinal, and cross-diagnostic and includes a comparison group of people from the general population who may be classified as "carers" but who are not caring for someone with special needs.

One proposition behind this work is that there are similarities in the experience of providing care across disability groups. At the same time, the experiences are likely to be different for carers of different ages and in different circumstances. The work covers a spectrum of ages and stages in carers and a range of disability groups. The research question is whether the disability, age, circumstances and other characteristics of the care recipient generally dominate, or whether the caregiver and environmental factors, and the ways in which services are provided, have at least an equal weight in determining the experience of caregiving. Obviously this is critical when considering changes in social policy.

Defining a Carer

Much of the past research uses stringent criteria for defining caregivers. For our purposes a carer could be a mother or a spouse providing 24-hours-a-day, 7-days-a-week care or a daughter, with her own family and work commitments, helping an aged parent with shopping or household chores for one hour or, for example, four days a week. It is our aim to explore the impact of caregiving on family caregivers in a wide variety of circumstances and levels of intensity of care. Therefore, caregivers are being selected on the basis of self-identification. The initial screening question asks whether the person has the main responsibility for providing care for someone who is aged or has a long-term illness, disability or other problem, even if living elsewhere. The non-carers are defined as people who are not caring for someone with special needs but who take primary responsibility for household tasks, including child care.

Measuring the Experience of Caregiving

While much investigation has concentrated on negative responses, or the burden of care, in general there is a recognition that people will experience similar situations in different ways. This has been described in the caregiver literature as a difference between objective and subjective burden (Hoenig and Hamilton 1966; Montgomery et al. 1985). The concept of objective burden is difficult by definition (Schene 1990). There is an assumption about the nature of the response to situations by the very use of the word burden. While the general point of interest when this concept is measured is the actual presence and frequency of particular behaviours or problem situations, this thinking limits the consideration of which factors are important in making the experience of caregiving burdensome or satisfying, and which affect the health and well-being of the caregiver.

The Social Behaviour Assessment Scale (Platt 1985) was developed with families of persons with schizophrenia and is designed as a comprehensive measure of subjective and objective burden. This separation into types of burden becomes irrelevant, however, if assessments are concerned with the overall sources of stress and coping.

Recent work has seen the preparation of a new range of instruments to assess the experience of caregiving. Instruments have been described which include positive dimensions (Kinney and Stephens 1989; Lawton et al. 1989) and a more complex assessment of the experience of caregiving (Pearlin et al. 1990; Ellis et al. 1989). These more comprehensive scales allow comparison with non-carers and the development of more effective research designs. The assessment of intervention strategies, for instance, requires sensitive measures of the caregivers' experience (Zarit 1989).

Instruments to assess the impact of care for dementia carers have been refined, with authors considering several dimensions of burden (Novak and Guest 1989) or of the consequences of caring (Pruchno and Potanishki 1989).

Based on their model of caregiving impact, Ellis et al. (1989) developed an instrument consisting of four major dimensions: caregiver involvement (with subscales related to assistance with activities of daily living), caregiver reactions (with subscales including impact on health, finances, social activities and so on); social support; and caregiver outcome (with subscales addressing positive well-being and depression). However, as the authors note, the instrument does not assess potentially positive reactions to caregiving.

With a substantial theoretical and empirical basis, Pearlin and colleagues (1990) developed a caregiver appraisal measure comprising 15 dimensions. These relate to "primary stressors" (derived from the needs of the care recipient and amount of care required), "secondary stressors" (additional demands and hardships generated by the primary stressors), and "mediating conditions" (factors which influence the caregiver's response to stress). While relatively comprehensive, with a strong theoretical basis and a high degree of face validity, the instrument focuses predominantly on the burdensome aspects of caregiving and is clearly developed for dementia caregiving.

Although still within the dementia literature, Braithwaite's (1992) needs-based concept of caregiving may provide a new direction for the development of instruments with a reduced emphasis on the negative aspects of caregiving and enhanced effectiveness in relation to the identification of interventions.

No instruments to date are ideal to assess broader aspects of the impact of care, or to consider which aspects are generic to caregiving, or specific to disorders within it. For the Carer's Programme, a broad assessment of the experience of providing care has been developed. This is a structured questionnaire which draws on items from existing scales and the literature about the various disability groups. In addition, exploratory interviews were conducted with small groups of carers to investigate their experience of caregiving. The aims of this exploratory work were to ensure that the researchers were closely in touch with the experiences and needs of family carers and, in this way, to assist in the development of an instrument which was comprehensive and minimised the possibility of omitting important questions, particularly in relation to policy development. Exploratory interviews were conducted with families caring for children and adults with physical and intellectual disabilities. The groups were convened mainly through support organisations and specialist services and were conducted as open, small group discussions from which transcripts were prepared and examined.

Measuring the Response to the Experience of Caregiving

In the Carers' Programme we are comparing those who are caregivers with those who are not, using indicators of health and well-being as outcome measures. The experience of care, as assessed above, and the activities of care, measured separately, may be regarded as independent variables. In this way, the experience of the caregiving role, positive and/or negative, becomes one of the variables used to predict overall health and well-being.

Measures of mental health are preferred to the identification of mental ill health, both because we are working with the underlying aim of promoting mental health in caregivers and because we are interested in measures which will be relatively sensitive to change. Mental health, when considered as satisfaction with life, happiness, feelings of well-being and self-fulfillment, is also intuitively more related to an assessment of the quality of life.

Attention to the possible confounding of independent and dependent variables is important in choosing the mental and physical health outcome measures. It is possible that trait depression and neuroticism predict the response to caregiving or contribute to response bias. There is also the potential for the relationship between caregiving and physical health to be confounded by trait negative affectivity. Self-report health measures have been said to reflect a pervasive mood disposition of negative affectivity (Watson and Pennebaker 1989).

In the Carers' Programme we are using indicators of mental and physical well-being as outcome measures. The use of repeated measures will allow us to assess the possible confounding effects of trait characteristics. Mental well-being is measured by the Positive and Negative Affect Scale (PANAS) of Watson et al. (1988). Physical health is measured with a questionnaire about health-related behaviours: number of visits to a doctor or a health centre, time in hospital, and use of medications, over a period of a year. A short measure of life satisfaction is used (Headey and Wearing 1981).

Conceptual Framework for the Study

Since the focus of interest in the Carers' Programme is the impact of the experience of the role of caregiver on mental and physical well-being, the framework of the study needs to relate to other studies of the determinants of mental health and well-being. Given that the experience of caregiving is usually thought of as "burden" and "stress," the cognitive theory of psychological stress and coping (Folkman et al. 1986) is particularly relevant. This approach has been used by investigators focussing on carers for the elderly (Pearlin et al. 1990; Ellis et al. 1989; Haley 1983; Zarit et al. 1986; Pratt et al. 1986; Quayhagen and Quayhagen 1988; Barusch 1988). This theoretical approach allows the comparison of caregivers and non-caregivers and also encourages the identification of those strategies which caregivers use to minimise the negative impact and to maximise the positive impact that caregiving has on their mental and physical well-being. The identification of such strategies will be of interest in understanding the dynamic aspects of the quality of life of caregivers.

Despite an extensive body of research into the effects of informal caregiving in the home, the literature is characterised by lack of agreement on significant findings. This probably reflects the lack of theoretical or methodological uniformity in the studies. The variables which have been most frequently measured are shown in Figure 1. This figure proposes a model of the relationship between variables relevant to the studies, within a stress and coping framework. The model is at a preliminary stage of development and will need refinement as data become available for analysis.

The relationship between the measure of the experience of care and the selected indicators of well-being will be explored at a simple level before mediating variables are brought into the model.

Caregiver characteristics	Care recipient characteristics
Sex	Sex
Age	Age
Employment status	Relationship to carer
Ethnicity	Income
Education	Tasks requiring assistance
Income	Diagnosed condition
Caregiving situation	**Cognitive/affective response to caregiving role**
Activities performed	Attitudes to/knowledge of diagnosed condition
Duration of Care	Perceived ability of care recipient
Financial costs	Attribution of behaviour control
Frequency of problems	Value given to caring role
Behaviours	General experience or role
Accommodation	

Possible mediating variables

Premorbid relationship with caregiver
Social supports of caregiver
Social supports of care recipient
Knowledge and use of formal services
Informal assistance received
Coping strategies/resources
Desire for institutionalization

Mental and Physical Health

State positive/negative affect
Physical health behaviours
Life satisfaction

Fig. 1 Modelling the experience and impact of caregiving

A Pilot Study: Methods and Results

The questionnaire developed to identify and obtain information from special needs carers and the comparison group of general carers was used in an initial study in Melbourne in November 1992. Using the Australian Institute of Family Studies' Computer Assisted Telephone Interviewing System and a team of trained interviewers, a state wide random survey of 2000 telephone numbers was conducted.

Caregivers were identified by responding "yes" to the question, "Do you have the main responsibility for someone who is aged or has a long-term illness, disability or other problem, even if they live elsewhere?" The comparison group was randomly selected from households where there was *no* main caregiver or a person with disabilities identified. In these households the person who took primary responsibility for housework and/or child care was selected for interview. The aim was to obtain a comparison group which was socio-demographically similar to our caregiver sample. Selected questions from the main caregiver interview, including those relating to sociodemographic characteristics, responsibility for household tasks, social support, health and emotional well-being, were asked of the comparison group.

Response Rate

Excluding 305 telephone numbers which were found to be disconnected, non-residential or non-contactable (engaged or not anwered on repeated occasions), 91% of contacted households were screened; that is, 9% refused to answer screening questions. Of the 136 caregivers identified, 72% agreed to be interviewed. The response rate for the comparison group was a slightly lower 68%. The proportion of households in which a carer was identified was calculated at 9%.

Findings

Socio-Demographic Characteristics and Household Responsibilities

Not surprisingly women predominated in each group. Caregivers covered a wide spectrum of ages but, consistent with other research, most fell in the middle age ranges, with over 70% in each group aged between 30 and 59 years. Most (over three quarters) were married.

The overwhelming majority in each group (80% of carers and 74% of the comparison group), as in the general population of Victoria (77% in the 1986 ABS Census), were Australian born. Neither did they differ in relation to employment status or educational qualifications: around half in each group (54% of carers and 47% of the comparison group) were not in paid employment, and similar proportions had no post-school qualifications (54% of carers and 52% of the comparison group).

The chi square statistic was used to test for statistically significant differences between the carers and the comparison group on a range of socio-demographic variables. There were no statistically significant differences between the two groups in relation to sex, age distribution or marital status (Table 1).

The similarity between our special needs carers and comparison group carers extended into childcare and household responsibilities. There were no statistically significant differences between the two groups in the number of children in the household, although carers were marginally less likely to be caring for children than were the comparison group (55% of carers compared with 43% of the comparison group).

Other variables on which the two groups did not significantly differ were income, the importance of religion, and whether they had been a carer in the past or were likely to be in the future.

The high degree of similarity between the special needs carers and the comparison carers on a variety of socio-demographic measures and in relation to household responsibilities and child care indicates the effectiveness of our method of selecting the comparison group.

The caregivers were a diverse group in terms of relationship to the care recipient, residential status, duration of care, time spent caring and the attributes of the care recipient (Schofield and Herrman 1993). Most were mothers,

Table 1. Characteristics of carers

	Carers n = 98 (%)	Comparison group n = 80 (%)
Sex		
Female	79	81
Male	21	19
Age in years		
15–29	6	14
30–44	40	51
45–59	33	23
60 and over	21	13
Marital status		
Married	77	75
Living with a partner	4	1
Neither	19	24
Country of origin		
Australia	80	74
Other English-speaking	9	7
Non-English speaking	11	19
Employment status		
Full time	27	33
Part time	19	20
Not in paid employment	54	47
Highest level of schooling		
No schooling – Year 8	19	17
Year 9–10	29	28
Year 11	24	14
Year 12	29	42
Post school qualifications		
None	54	52
Trade/apprenticeship	4	9
Tertiary qualification	20	18
Other qualification	22	21

daughters or spouses, but some were fathers, sons, grandchildren, siblings, daughters-in-law or friends. They were mostly living with the person for whom they cared (54%) or were caring for a relative who lived alone (22%). Some had been caring for only a few months but for most it was years, even decades. Carers differed, too, in the amount of time spent caring, but for the majority it was 7 days a week.

Not only was there diversity of carers but also of care recipients. They ranged in age from four to 98 years of age, but almost half were 75 years old or more. They represented a wide range of conditions including diabetes, stroke, dementia, heart disease, cancer, arthritis, asthma, musculoskeletal problems, psychiatric problems and intellectual disability. Most had multiple problems.

Use of formal services was low. Excluding carers whose relative was in residential care, only a minority of carers received regular formal services to assist in their caring role. The most frequently used services were transportation (e.g., community bus or multi-purpose taxis) and general home help, both of which were used by only 17% of carers. Specific home help, that is, assistance with minding, bathing or tasks specific to individual needs, was used by 12% of carers, with a similar proportion using community nursing services. Less than half (47%) of the carers had received any information about relevant services and organisations.

Social Support and Carer Overload

Participants were asked about the support they received from family and friends. The social support measures consisted of a three-item family support scale (Family), a five-item support from friends scale (Friends) and a two-item "esteemed by family and friends" scale (Esteem). The items were drawn from an existing measure (Turner et al. 1983) and factor analysis was used to identify broad dimensions. Mean scale scores were computed for each measure; respective alpha reliabilities coefficients for each measure are reported in Table 2 and indicate each scale's good internal consistency.

Differences between the carer and comparison samples in perceived social support on each of the three scales were assessed by t-tests for independent samples. Consistent with past research, these analyses revealed no statistically significant differences between the two groups in perceived social support from family or friends or in relation to others' estimation of one's competence (Esteem; Table 3).

The two groups were also compared on feelings of "overload." Overload was assessed by a three-item measure rated on a five-point Likert scale (Pearlin et al. 1990). Mean scale scores were computed and respective alpha coefficients for the carer and comparison samples were 0.77 and 0.73, indicating the scale's good internal consistency (Table 2). Again, differences between the two groups were assessed by t-tests for independent samples revealing no statistically significant difference between carers and the comparison group in relation to overload (Table 3).

Pertinently, the factors which did differentiate between our special needs caregivers and comparison carers were in relation to their own health and personal life satisfaction.

Carer Health

In relation to health status, there were statistically significant differences between the two groups (Table 4). More than twice the proportion of special needs carers as general carers reported having major health problems over the past 12 months (42% compared with 20% of the comparison group; chi square = 9.65, $p < 0.01$) and a long-term illness or disability (33% compared with 15%; chi square = 7.38, $p < 0.01$). Most commonly noted were asthma,

Table 2. Internal consistency (alpha) coefficients for life satisfaction, carer overload, three social support measures, positive and negative affect

	Carer sample		Comparison sample	
	Alpha	n	Alpha	n
Life satisfaction scale[a]	0.82	96	0.77	71
Your personal/emotional life				
Your life as a whole				
Your independence or freedom				
The respect and recognition you get				
Your health				
Your opportunities for leisure or recreation				
The amount of time you have to do the things you want to do				
The help you receive around the house				
Carer overload[b]	0.77	94	0.73	80
I'm exhausted when I go to bed at night				
I have more things to do than I can handle				
I don't have time for myself				
Social support scales[b]				
Family	0.75	97	0.60	80
Sometimes I'm not so sure if I can completely rely on family				
No matter what happens, I know that my family will always be there for me should I need them				
I know my family will always stand by me				
Friends	0.75	97	0.66	80
I have at least one friend I could tell anything to				
When I want to go out and do things I know that many of my friends would enjoy doing these things with me				
Even when I'm with my friends I feel alone				
When I'm with my friends I feel completely able to relax and be myself				
Esteem	2.68	97	0.61	80
People who know me think I'm good at what I do				
People in my family have confidence in me				
PANAS[c]				
Positive affect	0.81	93	0.79	78
Negative affect	0.88	93	0.83	79

[a] Items were rated on a five-point scale (very satisfied = 1, satisfied = 2, not sure = 3, dissatisfied = 4, very dissatisfied = 5)
[b] Items were rated on a five-point scale (strongly agree = 1, agree = 2, not sure = 3, disagree = 4, strongly disagree = 5)
[c] Items were rated on a five-point scale (not at all = 1, a little = 2, moderately = 3, quite a bit = 4, extremely = 5)

Table 3. Life satisfaction, carer overload, social support, PANAS: comparison of mean scale scores

	Carer	Comparison group	t-value	p<
Life satisfaction				
Mean	2.42	2.20	−2.23	0.05
SD	0.699	0.567		
n	96	80		
Carer overload				
Mean	2.79	2.95	1.09	ns
SD	1.003	0.911		
n	98	80		
Social support				
Family				
Mean	2.17	2.03	−1.15	ns
SD	0.877	0.743		
n	97	80		
Friends				
Mean	1.92	2.07	1.73	ns
SD	0.631	0.531		
n	80	98		
Esteem				
Mean	1.86	1.95	1.04	ns
SD	0.569	0.543		
n	80	98		
PANAS				
Positive affect				
Mean	3.12	3.07	−0.48	ns
SD	0.721	0.702		
n	96	78		
Negative affect				
Mean	1.82	1.79	−0.37	ns
SD	0.750	0.651		
n	95	79		

SD, Standard deviation; ns, not significant

high blood pressure, back trouble, arthritis, migraines, bowel problems, kidney disease, diabetes, cancer, coronary disease, and stroke.

However, carers did not differ significantly from the comparison group in ratings of their overall health, with 25% of caregivers and a marginally higher 35% of the comparison group rating their health as excellent. Neither did they differ significantly in the proportions who felt hindered by health troubles; in each group, almost 80% denied that health problems stopped them doing the things they wanted to do.

Table 4. Reported health status percentages of carers and comparison group

		Carers n = 98	Comparison group n = 80	Chi	p<
Percentages having health problems	Yes	42	20	9.65	0.01
	No	58	80		
Percentages having a long-term disability	Yes	33	15	7.38	0.01
	No	67	85		
Percentages rating their own overall health as:	Excellent	25	35		ns
	Good	45	42		
	Fair/Poor	30	25		
Percentages indicating health troubles stop them doing the things they want to do	Yes, a lot	8	10		ns
	A little	12	12		
	No	78	80		

Life Satisfaction

Participants were asked about their satisfaction with various aspects of their life, including health, independence, opportunities for leisure, help they received around the house, and respect and recognition accorded to them (Headey and Wearing 1981). The measure was adapted from a scale developed in Melbourne and comprised eight items which participants were asked to rate on a five-point Likert scale ranging from very satisfied to very dissatisfied. Mean scales scores were computed. High alpha coefficients for each sample (0.82 for carers and 0.77 for comparison group, respectively) indicate the scale's good internal consistency (Table 2).

Differences between carers and the comparison group in reported life satisfaction were assessed by a t-test for independent samples (Table 3). Carers reported significantly less satisfaction with their lives than did the comparison group; mean scales scores were 2.42 and 2.20, respectively ($t = 2.23$, $p < 0.05$; on the life satisfaction scale a higher score equals less satisfaction).

Psychological well-being was measured by the 10-item positive and negative affect mood scales. The scales are brief and easy to administer, and substantial to high positive correlations have been reported between the negative affect scale and the Hopkins Symptoms Checklist, Beck Depression Inventory and STAI State Anxiety Scale (Watson et al. 1988). Alpha reliabilities for the positive and negative affect scales, which demonstrate high internal consistency, are reported in Table 2. T-tests for independent samples revealed no statistically significant differences between the two groups (Table 3).

In summary, it seems from our bivariate analyses that special needs carers are not only highly similar to our comparison carers in relation to socio-demographic characteristics and responsibility for household chores, but also in relation to feelings of overload as well as perceived support from family and friends. Variables which did differentiate between the two groups, however, were relatively objective measures of health status and life satisfaction defined in relatively concrete terms. Some multivariate analyses were undertaken to explore factors that contribute to variations in these major outcome variables.

Predicting Major Health Problems

As there was a non-significant trend for special needs carers to be older than the comparison carers, a discriminant function analysis was used to test the hypothesis that the observed differences in health status might be explained by differences in age. The aim of a discriminant function analysis is to establish and appropriately weight a set of variables to best predict membership of a group; in this case, having major health problems in the past 12 months. With the combined data from the carer and the comparison group samples, a discriminant function analysis to predict major health problems was undertaken. Variables included in the analysis were age, sex, education level, overload, the three social support measures, importance of religion and carer status (that is, special needs or comparison group).

Using Rao's stepwise method, three variables were selected for entry into the equation on the basis of their discriminating power. In order of entry these were carer status, level of education and overload (Table 5). Thus, being a special needs carer emerged as the most powerful predictor of reporting major health problems in the past year, followed by lower educational level and feelings of overload. The fact that age did not emerge as a significant predictor suggests that the higher incidence of perceived health problems in special needs caregivers is not explained by age-related morbidity.

Predicting Life Satisfaction

A multiple regression analysis was used to explore factors predicting lower life satisfaction. Factors entered into the equation were sex, age, employment status, educational level, number of children, number of household tasks, three social support measures, overload, importance of religion and carer status.

Table 5. Discriminant function analysis for predicting major health problems (n = 177)

	Discriminant function coefficients
Being a carer	0.65
Educational level (low)	0.52
Overload (high)	0.52

Percentages of cases correctly classified = 65%
Canonical correlations = 0.34

In order of importance, feelings of high overload, little support from family and friends and being a carer emerged in the statistically significant equation predicting lower levels of life satisfaction (beta values = 0.44, 0.28, 0.17 and 0.15, respectively; multiple $R = 0.68$, $F = 10.28$, $p < 0.001$). The remaining variables did not contribute to the predictive equation at the level of statistical significance.

Predicting Feelings of Overload

As high overload was the most powerful predictor of diminished life satisfaction, a multiple regression analysis was also used to explore factors contributing to variations in feelings of overload. Variables entered into the equation were sex, age, employment status, educational level, number of children, number of household tasks, three social support measures, positive and negative affect, importance of religion and carer status. In order of importance, high negative affect, caring for a larger number of children and having the responsibility for a greater number of household tasks emerged as the significant predictors of high overload (beta values = 0.23, 0.23, 0.22, respectively; multiple $R = 50$, $F = 4.13$, $p < 0.001$). The remaining variables did not significantly contribute to the predictive equation.

Discussion

Using self-identification as the method of recruiting carer participants in this statewide random survey without imposing arbitrary exclusion criteria resulted in the inclusion of a broad diversity of carers. Carers were not only diverse in terms of age, sex, and relationship to care recipient but also in the amount of time spent caring and the number of activities of daily living for which help was given. Notwithstanding these differences within the carer sample, which may imply varying levels of intensity of care, are there differences between carers of people with disabilities and the comparison group, the latter being carers in the sense of taking primary responsibility for household tasks and/or child care?

Differences in outcome measures such as physical health and life satisfaction may vary according to a host of factors such as age, sex, employment or marital status. Hence it was the aim of this study to recruit a comparison group as similar to our carer sample as possible to minimize the confounding effects of such extraneous variables. Consistent with our aim, there was a high degree of similarity between the two groups in terms of sex and age distribution, ethnic background, educational level, marital status, employment status, and number of children as well as responsibility for household tasks.

However, on relatively objective measures of health status, that is, reported major health problems and chronic disability, there was a higher rate of ill-health among special needs carers than in the comparison group. This difference was not explained by age-related morbidity. Speculatively, the failure of the subjective health ratings to differentiate between the special needs and comparison carers, notwithstanding the self-reported objective differences, indicates a degree of stoicism on the part of special needs caregivers. Interestingly, in a recent study which focussed on elderly people with disabilities living in the community, Jorm et al. (1993) used one of the same subjective health ratings (that is, a single item health rating of excellent, good, fair and poor) to assess the physical health of carers. In a comparison with informants of elderly people who needed no help, subjective ill-health ratings were found to be significantly higher in carers of elderly people with physical disability, but no difference was found for behavioural disability.

The other major factor which differentiated between the special needs carers and the comparison group was diminished life satisfaction.

Looked at in isolation, and consistent with some studies in the past (Haley et al. 1987), perceived social support did not significantly differentiate between the carers and the comparison group; likewise with feelings of overload. However, in combination these factors mediated differences between the two groups on major outcome variables. In a study which considered whether social supports operated as a buffer or a stress, Fiore et al. (1983) found that negative ratings of social contacts predicted depression in their sample of spouse caregivers of partners with dementia. In the present study, feelings of overload linked with being a special needs carer to predict major health problems. High overload linked with feelings of low social support and being a special needs carer to predict diminished life satisfaction. In turn, feelings of anxiety and depression (negative affect) were linked with the burden of household chores and childcare to predict overload. It is important to note, however, that in these cross-sectional data it is not possible to attribute causal connections.

In spite of the diversity of special needs carers, covering a broad spectrum of caring roles, there were clear differences between this group and the comparison group of general carers in relation to health and well-being. Illness and disability were more common in carers of people with disabilities, particularly in carers who felt exhausted and unable to cope with the demands upon them. Likewise, diminished life satisfaction was more common in special needs carers, particularly in those who felt burdened by the demands upon them and less cushioned by family and friends.

This is a limited picture using only the small set of questions for which we have data from our comparison group. Findings relating to the particular demands placed on our carers – physical, emotional and financial, arising from the special needs of the care recipient – are yet to be analyzed. Obviously with the variety of caregiving roles and responses, a larger sample of carers is required to obtain a profile of carers in the state; to explore, for example, the interactive effects of gender, residential status, relationship, nature of disability, age of carer and care recipient on the effects of caring, and, most importantly, to identify carer needs and strategies for easing the pressures. On the basis of these early findings we are proceeding with a more extensive survey which will also form the base line for a follow-up study. We are encouraged that the self-report measures employed in this work are useful pointers to quality of life of the caregivers in our community. In the next phase of work we will be assessing this further in home-based interviews with sub-samples of the identified caregivers. Thus, this overall project will provide a comprehensive view of the characteristics of a community sample of caregivers.

References

Barusch HS (1988) Problems and coping strategies of elderly spouse caregivers. Gerontologist 28:677–685

Baumgarten M (1989) The health of persons giving care to the demented elderly: a critical review of the literature. Clin Epidemiol 42(12):1137–1148

Braithwaite V (1986) The burden of home care: how is it shared? Suppl Community Health Stud 10:7–11

Braithwaite V (1990) Bound to care. Sydney, Allen&Unwin

Braithwaite V (1992) Caregiving burden: making the concept scientifically useful and policy relevant. Res Ageing 14(1):3–27

Brodaty H, Gresham M (1989) Effect of a training programme to reduce stress in carers of patients with dementia. Brit Med J 299:1375–1379

Draper BM, Poulos CJ, Cole AMD, Poulos RG, Ehrlich F (1992) A comparison of caregivers for elderly stroke and dementia victims. J Am Geriat Soc 40:896–901

Dupont A (1986) Socio-psychiatric aspects of the young severely mentally retarded and the family. Brit J Psychiat 148:227–234

Ellis BH, Miller KI, Given SW (1989) Caregivers in home health care situations: measurement and relations among critical concepts. Health Commun 1(4):207–226

Fadden G, Bebbington P, Kuipers L (1987) The burden of care: the impact of functional psychiatric illness on the patient's family. Brit J Psychiat 154:768–775

Fiore J, Becker J, Coppel DB (1983) Social Network Interactions: A buffer or a stress. Am J Community Psychol 11:423–439

Fitting M, Rabins P, Lucas MJ, Eastham J (1986) Caregivers for dementia patients: comparison of husbands and wives. Gerontologist 26:248–252

Folkman S, Lazarus R, Gruen R, DeLongis A (1986) Appraisal, coping, health status and psychological symptoms. J Personality Soc Psychol 50:571–579

Gallagher D, Lovett S, Zeiss A (1989) Interventions with caregivers of frail elderly persons. In: Ory MG, Bond K (eds) Ageing and Health Care. London, Routledge, pp 167–190

Gibson D (1984) Knowledge of community services amongst the aged. Australian J Society Issues 19:3–13

Green H (1985) Informal carers. General Household Survey, 15, Supplement A, HMSO, London

Gwyther LP, George LK (1986) Caregivers for dementia patients: complex determinants of wellbeing and burden. Gerontologist 26:245–247

Haley WE (1983) A family-behavioural approach to the treatment of the cognitively impaired elderly. Gerontologist 23:18–20

Haley WE, Levine EG, Brown SL, Berry JW, Hughes GH (1987) Psychological, social and health consequences of caring for a relative with senile dementia. J Am Geriat Soc 35:405–411

Harper S, Lund DA (1990) Wives, husbands and daughters caring for institutionalized and non-institutionalized dementia patients: towards a model of caregiver burden. Internat J Aging Human Devel 30(4):241–262

Headey B, Wearing AJ (1981) Australians Priorities, Satisfactions and Wellbeing. University of Melbourne, Department of Community Welfare Service Monograph in Public Policy Studies No. 4

Herrman H, Singh B, Schofield H, Eastwood R, Burgess P, Lewis V. Scotton R (1993) The health and wellbeing of informal caregivers: a review and study programme. Australian J Public Health 17:261–266

Hoenig J, Hamilton MW (1966) The schizophrenic patient in the community and his effect on the household. Internat J Soc Psychiat 165–176

Hooyman NR, Kiyak HA (1991) Social Gerontology: a multidisciplinary perspective (2nd ed). Allyn and Bacon, Massachusetts

Horowitz A (1985) Sons and daughters as caregivers to older patients: difference in role performance and consequences. Gerontologist 25:612–617

Jorm AF, Henderson S, Scott R, MacKinnon AJ, Korten AE, Christensen H (1993) The disabled elderly living in the community: care received from family and formal services. Med J Australia 158:383–388

Jutras S, Veilleux F (1991) Informal caregiving: gender roles and care giving to the elderly: an empirical study. Sex Roles 25:1–18

Kinnear D, Graycar A (1984) Ageing and family dependency. Australian J Society Issues 19:13–26

Kinney JM, Stephens MAP (1989) Hassles and uplifts of giving care to a family member with dementia. Psychol Ageing 26:273–278

Lawton MP, Kleban MH, Moss M, Rovine M, Glicksman A (1989) Measuring caregiving appraisal. J Gerontol 44:61–67

Lefley HP (1987) Aging parents as caregivers of mentally ill adult children: an emerging social problem. Hospital Community Psychiat 38:1063–1070

Levin E, Sinclair I, Gorbach P (1989) Families, services and confusion in old age. Avebury, Hants

MacCarthy B, Lesage A, Brewin CR, Brugha TS, Mangen S, Wing JK (1989a) Needs for care among the relatives of long-term users of day care. Psychol Med 19:725–736

MacCarthy B, Kuipers L, Hurry J, Harper R, le Sage A (1989b) Counselling the relatives of the long-term adult mentally ill. I. Evaluation of the impact on relatives and patients. Brit J Psychiat 154:768–775

Montgomery RJV, Gonyea JC, Hooyman NR (1985) Caregiving and the experience of subjective and objective burden. Family Rel 34:19–25

Morris RG, Morris LW, Britton PG (1988) Factors affecting the emotional wellbeing of the caregivers of dementia sufferers. Brit J Psychiat 153:147–156

O'Connor DW, Pollitt PA, Hyde JB, Brook CPB, Reiss BB, Roth M (1988) Do general practitioners miss dementia in elderly patients? Brit Med J 297:1107–1110

Novak M, Guest C (1989) Caregiver response to Alzheimer's disease. Internat J Aging Human Develop 28:67–79

Pearlin LI, Mullan JT, Semple SJ, Skaff MM (1990) Caregiving and the stress process: An overview of concepts and their measures. Gerontologist 30(5):563–594

Platt S (1985) Measuring the burden of psychiatric illness on the family: an evaluation of some rating scales. Psychol Med 15:383–389

Pratt C, Schmall V, Wright S (1986) Family caregivers and dementia: social casework. J Contemporary Soc Work, 67:119–124

Pruchno RA, Potanishki SL (1989) Caregiving spouses: physical and mental health in perspective. J Am Geriat Soc 37:697–705

Quayhagen MP, Quayhagen M (1988) Alzheimer's stress: coping with the caregiving role. Gerontologist 28:391–396

Romans-Clarkson SE, Clarkson JE, Dittmen ID, Flett R, Linsell C, Mullen PE, Mullin B (1986) Impact of a handicapped child on mental health of parents. Brit Med J 293:1395–1397

Schene AH (1990) Objective and subjective dimensions of family burden: towards an integrated framework for research. Soc Psychiat Psychiat Epidemiol 25:289–297

Schofield H, Herrman H (1993) Characteristics of carers in Victoria. Family Matters (34):21–36

Schultz CL, Schultz NC (1990) Caring for family caregivers. Australian J Marriage Family 11:84–93

Sherman BR, Cocozza JJ (1984) Stress in families of the developmentally disabled: a literature review of factors affecting the decision to seek out-of-home placements. Family Relations 33(1):95–103
Smith JV, Birchwood MJ (1987) Specific and non-specific effects of education intervention with families living with a shizophrenic relative. Brit J Psychiat 150:645–652
Stone R, Cafferata GL, Sangl J (1987) Caregivers of the frail elderly: a national profile. Gerontologist 27:616–626
Trute B (1990) Child and parent predictors of family adjustment in households containing young developmentally disabled children. Family Relations 39(3):292–297
Turner D, Frankel BG, Lewin DM (1983) Social support: conceptualization, measurement and implication for mental health. Community Mental Health 3:67–111
Wasow M (1985) Chronic schizophrenia and spouses and children compared. J Chronic Disabilities 38:711–716
Watson D, Clark LA, Tellegen A (1988) Development and validation of brief measures of Positive and Negative Affect: The PANAS Scales. J Personality Soc Psychol 54: 1063–1070
Watson D, Pennebaker J (1989) Health complaints, stress and distress: exploring the central role of negative affectivity. Psychol Rev 96:234–254
Wells Y, Jorm AF (1987) Evaluation of a special nursing home unit for dementia sufferers: a randomised controlled comparison with community care. Australian New Zealand J Psychiat 21:524–531
Whittick JE (1988) Dementia and mental handicap: emotional distress in carers. Brit J Clin Psychol 27:167–172
Zarit SH, Todd PA, Zarit JM (1986) Subjective burden of husbands and wives as caregivers: a longitudinal study. Gerontologist 26:260–266
Zarit SH (1989) Issues and directions in family intervention research. In: Light E, Lebowitz BD (eds) Alzheimer's disease treatment and familiy stress: directions of research. US Department of Health and Human Services, Public Health Services, ADAMHA & NIMH, pp 458–486
Zarit S, Toseland R (1989) Current and future direction in family caregiving research. Gerontologist 29:481–483

Quality of Life Assessment in Arthritis

S. M. Skevington

Summary

Arthritis is rarely fatal but profoundly affects functioning, so there are important quality of life implications for these patients. Pain and disability are key issues in this disease, and has stimulated discussion of more general points on measuring quality of life cross-culturally. Following general remarks about conceptualization of the issue, this report reviews some important scales and concludes that, while a number of generic and specific instruments exist which could be used to evaluate the lives of those with arthritis, several do not assess pain and none includes the broad range of quality of life issues, positive and negative, to provide a comprehensive assessment. Future scales will need to take account of the fluctuating nature of the disease and how this affects the stability of measurement.

Introduction

Arthritis is widespread in the Western World (Scotch and Geiger 1962). It is estimated that between 5% and 7% of the population of North America and Britain are disabled by musculoskeletal conditions (Badley 1992). The Arthritis and Rheumatism Council of Great Britain report that only one person in 50 can expect to escape some form of rheumatic complaint during his/her lifetime.

Arthritis is also the most common cause of disability (Martin et al. 1988), having the potential for severely limiting activities. Of those who attend for treatment, about one quarter recover completely, another quarter heal but have slight residual joint damage which does not interfere with their work, 40% have continual disease activity but are not bedridden and, despite the image of the disease, only 10% are severely crippled (Jayson and Dixon 1980). Four ways in which rheumatic disease limits performance of duties and activities were categorised as early as 1949 (Steinbroker et al. 1949). They range from complete functional capacity to the total incapacity of being bedridden. The assessment of functional status has been recently revised to more profitably distinguish between self-care activities – like dressing and feeding, the vocational activities of schoolwork, homemaking and work – and avocational

J. Orley, W. Kuyken (Eds.)
Quality of Life Assessment:
International Perspectives

activities, such as recreation and leisure (Hochberg et al. 1992). Because of this concern, measures of functional status which often include a detailed assessment of activities of daily living have been widely developed for use specifically with these diseases.

Deyo (1988) observed that rheumatoid arthritis (RA) is a "prototypical chronic disease, as its impacts are largely functional and rarely fatal" (p 205). While not imminently life-threatening, RA may reduce the life span by about 10 years. RA is associated with significantly greater mortality than osteoarthritis (OA). Co-morbidity with other diseases is common in RA, with the highest levels among those with little formal education (Pincus and Callaghan 1986). Therefore arthritis patients could benefit greatly from the development of a reliable, valid and responsive quality of life measure which could comprehensively chart their needs. Osteoarthritis is a common cause of severe disabling intractable pain but, while some patients report severe pain, others are asymptomatic (Dieppe et al. 1989). Therefore joint pain is a sufficient but not a necessary feature in the diagnosis of arthritic disease (Ropes et al. 1958). Nevertheless pain is a "powerful motivator" (Melzack and Dennis 1978) and, for many people with arthritis, pain is the main symptom that brings them to treatment initially. However, this persistent search for relief may subsequently predispose patients to accept and persist with treatments which have undesirable side effects, and those in turn can influence the quality of life. The benefits of some treatments may well be outweighed by the physical side effects, psychological distress and decline in quality of life (Fallowfield 1990). Examples are the gastrointestinal disorders which affect nearly half of those treated with non-steroidal anti-inflammatory drugs (NSAIDS). Their intake results in haemorrhage and emergency hospital admission for an estimated 30,000 patients in UK annually (Jacyna 1992). While medical economists have estimated these "shadow costs" to the health budget in pounds Sterling, few seem to have counted the human cost to quality of life of the persistent indigestion and apprehension of long-term use, combined with the trauma of a life-threatening emergency and reduced expectations for successful future treatment. These costs are in addition to those of having the disease itself.

A special methodological problem which deserves attention in designing a quality of life scale for use by people with arthritis is that several aspects of the disease affect the stability of measurements over time. RA is known for its capricious nature and periodic "flares" alternating with relief. Furthermore there are considerable diurnal variations in pain and stiffness. Despite the general shortage of reliable scientific evidence in this area, subjective changes in pain associated with the weather and seasons are frequently reported and are believed to be important by many patients, so these beliefs may also affect measurement stability (Shutty, Lundiff and De Good 1992).

Some Conceptual Issues

While many aspects of quality of life affected by arthritis have been identified using a variety of quantitative and qualitative methods, Deyo (1988) pointed out that the overriding concern of those who consult is to be free of pain and to be able to perform their accustomed activities. As a rule patients do not care about their erythrosedimentation rate (ESR), titre of rheumatoid factor or activity on the joint scan. This attitude is perhaps as well, as many of these key clinical diagnostic measures are unreliable. For instance, two ESR results taken from the same observer or the same laboratory can show 20% variability, and other examples are provided in Deyo's table (see Table 1). However, many researchers place great emphasis on the use of these "objective" measures, claiming that they are more reliable than subjective ones. Such confidence in these measures is patently unwarranted in the arthritic diseases, at least.

The proliferation of profiles and indices in the search for a comprehensive and psychometrically sound quality of life measure reflects the widespread dissatisfaction with existing forms and indicates that a new approach to the conceptualization of quality of life is urgently needed. Where subjective measures of quality of life have been developed to enable patients to evaluate their own condition, assessment has often been restricted to areas of direct medical concern, such as symptoms and disability, without much taking account of the broader qualities of life. Calman (1987) sees quality of life not only in terms of those dimensions pertaining to physical problems and psychosocial and spiritual factors, which frequently form the major content of many instruments, but he also describes a range of wider dimensions which are rarely considered, such as individual ambitions, priorities and accomplishments, cultural aspects, timing, politics and an individual's philosophy. Some generic measures like the Sickness Impact Profile (Bergner et al. 1981) provide a more intricate multidimensional approach to the concept but still fall short of encom-

Table 1. Relevance and reliability of various outcome measures for arthritis trials[a]

Type	Measures	Estimated patient relevance	Estimated variability (same laboratory or observer)
Laboratory	Sedimentation rate (ESR)	0	20%
	Latex fixation titre	0	2 tubes
	Haemoglobin	+	5%
Surrogate measures of outcome	Grip strength	+	20%
	Walking	+	20%
	Patient global assessment	+ +	1 grade
True outcome measures	Disability	+ + + +	7%
	Physical discomfort	+ + + +	15%
	Financial impact	+ + + +	10%

[a] From Deyo (1988)

passing the wide-ranging issues which Calman deems to be important. Recently there has been a call for investigators to return to basics by collecting qualitative information to reassess the number of basic dimensions which comprise quality of life (Bowling 1993). The methodology used to design the WHOQOL has made a genuine contribution in this direction.

It would be fair to say that many positive aspects of quality of life have been badly neglected in most assessments. The style of their design is conceptually driven by the pathology of the clinic and the problem-oriented approach presented by patients and adopted by clinicians as part of their respective roles. This means that the content of a clinical interview for those with arthritis is inevitably focussed on the amelioration of pain, inflammation and immobility, which have profound consequences for the lives of patients. But any comprehensive assessment of quality of life must necessarily take the positive aspects of people's lives into account if a holistic view is to be generated. The misery of chronic arthritis may be seen as being balanced and even compensated by a close family life, the joys of singing in a choir and the pleasures of good burgundy for instance, so it seems mistaken to give precedence to merely one half of this concept.

Rarely do quality of life measures include even a nodding acquaintance with the positive affect of happiness, for instance. In re-evaluating the concept of happiness, Ryff (1989) identified six important and stable aspects. These were self-acceptance, positive relations with others, autonomy, environmental mastery, personal growth and purpose in life. These aspects should be actively incorporated into any generic assessment. Furthermore, for some, having a chronic illness may paradoxically help to develop a more positive side to life.

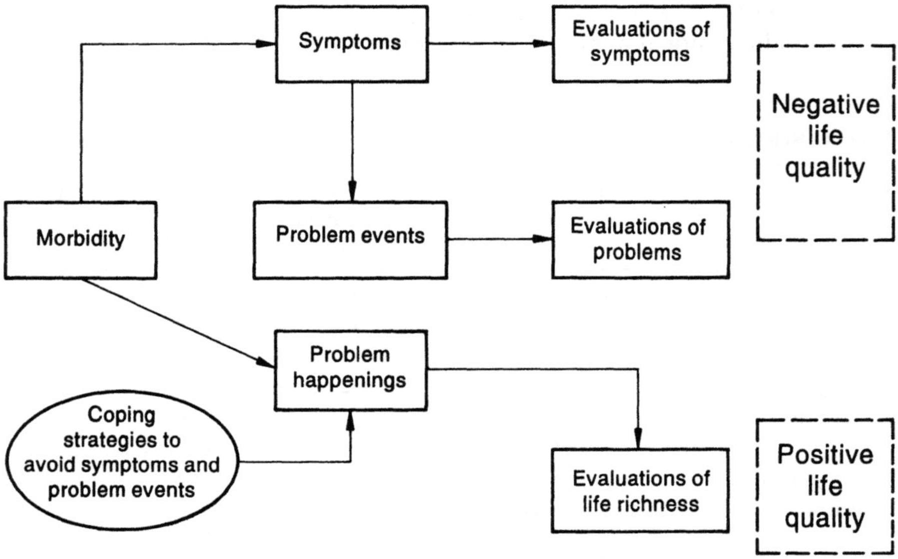

Fig. 1 Different causal sequences for positive and negative life quality. From Hyland (1992)

As a result of their pain and illness, those with arthritis sometimes learn new ways of doing things, such as opening a can or driving the car, and this new knowledge may have an enriching effect on their lives rather than detracting from them, depending on individual interpretation. Interviews with arthritis patients reveal that they do discover new strengths as a result of their illness, sometimes in an infinitely resourceful way, and this personal growth and greater autonomy are key facets of happiness (Skevington 1994). Hyland (1992) elaborated this idea in a recent model of different causal sequences for positive and negative quality of life events (see Fig. 1).

Few existing scales and indices provide a means of assessing the patient's priorities for a good life. In the study of arthritis exceptions to this are the MACTAR (Tugwell et al. 1987) and AIMS 2 (Meenan et al. 1992). Not only do we need to know which aspects of life are the most and least important but also which ones people might want to change and what their priorities might be for changing them. None of these issues can be assumed but, in the daily life of clinics, these priorities have tended to be assumed by health professionals using clinical intuition. So a method which provides the treater with a record of the patient's priorities and desires for change serves a useful clinical purpose. New methods of statistical analysis may be needed to tackle this problem in a satisfactory way.

Cross-Cultural Issues

The importance of designing scales which can evaluate quality of life in chronic illness cross-culturally has been raised by Sartorius (1987, 1993). There are broad-ranging cultural differences in health and illness behaviour and in the presentation of the sick role, which complicate comparisons of health assessments. Geddes (1985) has pointed out that an unpleasantness which is common in a society often tends to be devalued, so that cough, sputum and breathlessness are largely ignored in the poorer industrial communities of northern England, whereas in Nigeria malaria is so common it equates with the English cold.

As pain is central to the study of quality of life in arthritis, this symptom provides a useful illustration of several pertinent cross-cultural issues likely to be encountered in its assessment. Modern psycho-physical methods have shown that sensation thresholds are similar universally and do not distinguish reliably between ethnic groups. But the point at which people begin to report pain and how much they are inclined to tolerate are profoundly affected by social and cultural factors. In a study of Nepalese sherpas, Clark and Clark (1980) found they were far more stoical than the Europeans with whom they were working. The porters were prepared to receive much higher levels of electrical stimulation than their Western companions before describing them as painful. This further justifies the necessity of grappling with the difficult problem of cross-cultural differences in subjective pain reports (Zborowski 1952; Zola 1966). However, in addition to interethnic differences, substantial intraethnic heterogeneity has been recorded in the ways pain is experienced and reported, as an investigation of seven ethnic groups in New York has shown (Lipton and Marbach 1984). One strength of the WHOQOL methodology is that it would be capable of accommodating and assessing this feature in addition to more widely expected interethnic differences.

There are likely to be problems in choosing universal words to describe pain, given the diversity of cultural concepts and meanings associated with pain. Looking at the language of pain, Fabrega and Timms (1976) observed that English has four basic words for pain – pain, hurt, sore and ache – whereas the Japanese language has three and Thai only two. Equating and weighting these items alone would not easily enable cross-cultural comparisons, even with the assistance of good translation and back-translation facilities. Hunt and colleagues (1986) catalogued the extensive problems associated with translating existing scales like the Sickness Impact Profile (SIP; Bergner et al. 1981) and the Nottingham Health Profile (NHP; Hunt et al. 1986) Graphically summarising in a discussion of the translation of the NHP for Arabic use they say: "... the conceptual world of an Egyptian peasant scarcely encompasses the daily health concerns of an English citizen or vice versa, and the exigencies of everyday life in rural Egypt can hardly be compared to those of an English town" (p 216).

The dual aim of achieving conceptual as well as semantic equivalence of two versions of the same scale has been confounded by this insurmountable methodological problem until very recently; the WHOQOL has progressed thinking here.

Quality of Life Instruments for Arthritis

In taxonomising quality of life scales, Guyatt and colleagues (1989) identified the strengths and weaknesses of generic and specific instruments. Both types have been used in the study of quality of life in arthritis, but how far do they assess the two main complaints of pain and disability which Deyo says are central to the concerns of arthritis patients?

Some scales were specifically designed to examine functional activities rather than the health status which is embraced by the much broader quality of life concept. There are several scales which examine up to 100 activities of daily living within this brief, using self-report and/or physician assessment. The best of these is probably the Functional Status Index (FSI), which also includes a measure of pain (Jette 1980). Separate versions for self-assessment and the treating physician acknowledge differing social perceptions of quality of life. The scale evaluates (on a scale from 0 to 4) the three dimensions of pain, dependence and difficulty (which are important in treatment outcomes) in performing 18 activities of daily living. While limited in scope to functional activity, this scale is reasonably reliable and valid and takes up to 30 minutes to be administered by a professional.

Another scale along similar lines is the Health Assessment Questionnaire (HAQ; Fries et al. 1980), which assesses difficulties with eight types of activity over the past week, with the use of aids and devices, and includes a Visual Analogue Scale (VAS) to measure pain intensity. The FSI appears to be more efficient than the HAQ (Liang et al. 1985), both overall and for pain, and so may be the most useful of the scales available for examining pain and activity.

VAS scales themselves are frequently used in studies of quality of life in arthritis to measure pain intensity e.g., a 100 mm line from no pain (0) to pain as bad as it could be (100). Intrinsic to the VAS design is the assumption that pain is a unidimensional experience, despite substantial evidence to the contrary in the pain literature. The qualities of the VAS for use with arthritic groups are well documented (Huskisson 1983), and the VAS has been used alone and in combination with other approaches. However, it has proved difficult to use, especially with respondents who are not literate and who also appear to have difficulty in understanding what is required numerically. In a Brazilian study, 91 RA patients completed three assessments of a 100 mm VAS from no pain to worst possible pain, a verbal rating scale (VRS) where five independent boxes were separately labelled between the two extremes, and a numerical rating scale (NRS) where 10 linked boxes like a row of bricks were numbered and labelled. A comparison of non-literates (n = 25) and literates showed that the NRS had the highest reliabilities for both groups (Ferraz et al. 1990).

While the McMaster Toronto Arthritis Patient Preference Disability Questionnaire (MACTAR; Bowling 1993) does not include pain as a direct measure, it presents a new approach to the investigation of activities, by asking RA patients to prioritise activities affected directly by inflammation. It then follows up by asking "which of these activities would you most like to do," thereby enabling patients to rank their disabilities and goals and to make comparisons later. This customised approach has the advantage that only activities relevant to pain and inflammation are assessed, but comparisons between patients and between groups are more difficult when dealing with small numbers. Other researchers have raised questions about the viability of goal-setting procedures; for example, in an unpublished clinical trial of housebound arthritics, 50% were unable to state a functional goal (Liang et al. 1982).

The Arthritis Impact Measurement Scale (AIMS; Meenan et al. 1980, 1982) directly incorporates the WHO definition of health as "physical, mental and social well-being" into its design. As is common in this area, it draws on items from previous scales. Pain forms one of nine subscales incorporating four of the 45 self-administered multi-choice questions designed in Guttman format. Overall validity and reliability are good (Cronbach's alpha for the pain subscale = 0.85). However, the accuracy of pain memories as long as one month ago seems questionable. The inclusion of the concept of stiffness with pain in the wording of this subscale is both unusual and desirable. The importance given to morning stiffness in diagnosis suggests that this symptom should be included in any specific measure. While the standardisation properties of the AIMS are good, a recent short-form version shows excellent properties, too (Wallston et al. 1989).

However, with the AIMS2 (Meenan et al. 1992), the original has been refined by removing insensitive and relatively unreliable items and by adding three new scales of arm function, work and social support. Conceptually more important are the added new assessments which enable respondents to show, for each area of health, how satisfied they have been, the impact of arthritis on each area and which three areas the patient believes are most in need of improvement. These changes go some way toward meeting some of the criticisms levelled at earlier instruments.

Conclusions

The best existing generic instruments have only assessed a very limited number of the many facets of quality of life and so, for arthritis as for other disorders and conditions, they fall short of being able to obtain a wholistic view of a person's total well-being. In particular, positive aspects of life such as happiness have been substantially neglected. Other scales such as the SF-36 lack Gestalt in piecing together psychometrically valid components and at the same time losing sight of the overall concept. The WHOQOL methodology will enable researchers to overcome the semantic and conceptual stumbling blocks they have faced in translating and back-translating existing scales. For these reasons the development of the WHOQOL provides a welcome advance in measurement.

References

Badley E (1992) The impact of musculoskeletal disorders on the Canadian population. Rheumtol 19:337–340

Bergner JM, Bobbitt RA, Carter WB, Gilson BS (1981) The Sickness Impact Profile: development and final revision of a health status measure. Med Care XIX (8):787–805

Bowling A (1993) Conceptual and measurement issues in identified dimensions of quality of life: social, psychological and physical. Paper to the Health Related Quality of Life Workshop, Society for Social Medicine, Sheffield

Calman KC (1987) Definitions and dimensions of quality of life. In: Aaronson NK, Beckman J (eds) The quality of life of cancer patients. Raven Press, New York, pp 1–9

Clark WB, Clark SB (1980) Pain responses in Nepalese porters. Science 209:410–412

Dieppe PA, Harkness JAL, Higgs ER (1989) Osteoarthritis. In: Wall PD, Melzack R (eds) Textbook of pain (second edition). Churchill Livingston, Edinburgh, pp 306–314

Deyo RA (1988) Measuring the quality of life of patients with rheumatoid arthritis. In: Walker SR, Rosser RM (eds) Quality of life: assessment and application. MTP Press, Lancaster, pp 205–222

Fabrega H, Timms S (1976) Culture, language and the shaping of an illness: an illustration based on pain. J Psychosomatic Res 20:323

Fallowfield L (1990) The quality of life: the missing measurement in health care. Souvenir Press, London.

Ferraz MB, Quaresma MR, Aquino LRL, Atra E, Tugwell P, Goldsmith CH (1990) Reliability of pain scales in the assessment of literate and illiterate patients with RA. J Rheumatol 17(8):1022

Fries J, Spitz P, Young D (1980) The dimensions of health outcomes: the Health Assessment Questionnaire, disability and pain scales. J Rheumatol 9:789–793
Geddes DM (1985) Quality of life. Clinics Oncol 4(1):161
Guyatt GH, van Zanten SJOV, Feeny DH, Patrick DL (1989) Measuring quality of life in clinical trials: a taxonomy and review. CMAJ 140:1441–1447
Hochberg MC, Chang RW, Dwosh I, Lindsey S, Pincus T, Wolfe F (1992) The American College of Rheumatology 1991 revised criteria for the classification of global functional status in Rheumatoid Arthritis. Arth Rheumat 35(5):498
Hunt SM, McEwan J, McKenna SP (1986) Cross-cultural issues in health indicators. Chapter 8. In: Measuring health status. Croom Helm, London, pp 203–224
Huskisson EC (1983) Visual Analogue Scales. In: Melzack R (ed) Pain measurement and assessment. Raven Press, New York, pp 33–37
Hyland M (1992) A reformulation of quality of life for medical science. Quality of Life Res 1:267–272
Jacyna M (1992) Serious gastrointestinal adverse events to NSAIDS: complications in the treatment of arthritis. Brit J Med Econ: An evaluation of the cost of arthritis 15:15–21
Jayson MIV, Dixon A StJ (1980) Rheumatism and Arthritis: What you should know about the problems and treatment. Pan, London
Jette AM (1980) Functional Status Index: reliability of a chronic disease evaluation instrument. Arch Phys Med Rehab 61:395–401
Liang MH, Cullen K, Larson M (1982) In search of a more perfect mousetrap (health status or quality of life instrument). J Rheumatol 9(5):775
Liang MH, Larson M, Cullen K, Schwartz JA (1985) Comparative measurement efficiency and sensitivity of five health status instruments for arthritis research. Arth Rheumat 28(5):542–547
Lipton JA, Marbach JJ (1984) Ethnicity and the pain experience. Soc Sci Med 19(12): 1279–1298
Martin J, Meltzer H, Elliott D (1988) The prevalence of disability among adults. HMSO London
Meenan RF, Gertman PM, Mason JH (1980) Measuring health status in arthritis: the Arthritis Impact Measurement Scales. Arth Rheumat 23(2):146–152
Meenan RF, Gertman PM, Mason JH, Dunaif R (1982) The Arthritis Impact Measurement Scales: further investigations of a health status measure. Arth Rheumat 25(9): 1048–1053
Meenan RF, Mason JH, Anderson JJ, Guccione AA, Kazis LE (1992) The content and properties of a revised and expanded Arthritis Impact Measurement Scales health status questionaire. Arthritis Rheumat 35(1):1–10
Melzack R, Dennis SC (1978) Neurophysiological foundations of pain. In: Sternbach RA (ed) The psychology of pain, Raven Press, New York, pp 1–26
Pincus T, Callaghan LF (1986) Taking mortality in Rheumatoid Arthritis seriously – predictive markers, socio-economic status and comorbidity. J Rheumatol 13(5):841–845
Ropes MW, Bennett GA, Cobb S, Jacox R, Jessar RA (1958) Revision of diagnostic criteria for Rheumatoid Arthritis. Arthritis and Rheumatism Foundation. Bull Rheumat Dis IX(4):175–176
Ryff CD (1989) Happiness is everything, or is it? Explorations on the meaning of the psychological well-being. J Personality Social Psychol 57(6):1069–1081
Sartorius N (1987) Cross-cultural comparisons of data about quality of life: a sample of issues. In: Aaronson NK, Beckman J (eds) The quality of life of cancer patients: Monographs of the European Organisation for research on the Treatment of Cancer (EORTC). Raven Press, New York, pp 19–24
Sartorius N (1993) WHO method for assessment of health-related quality of life. In: Walker SR, Rosser RM (eds) Quality of life assessment: key issues in the 1990's. Kluwer Academic Publishers, Dordrecht, Netherlands
Scotch NA, Geiger HJ (1962) The epidemiology of rheumatoid arthritis – a review with special attention to social factors. J Chron Dis 15:1037–1067

Shutty MS, Lundiff G, De Good DE (1992) Pain complaints and the weather: weather sensitivity and symptom complaints in chronic pain. Pain 49:199–204

Skevington SM (1994) Social comparisons in cross-cultural quality of life assessment. International Journal of Mental Health. Monograph on Quality of Life (in press)

Steinbroker O, Traeger C, Batterman R (1949) Therapeutic criteria in Rheumatoid Arthritis. JAMA 262:907–1013

Tugwell P, Bombardier C, Buchanan WW, Goldsmith CH, Grace E, Hanna B (1987) The MACTAR patient preference disability questionnaire – an individual functional priority approach for assessing improvement in physical disability in clinical trials in Rheumatoid Arthritis. J Rheumatol 14(3):446–451

Wallston KA, Brown GK, Stein MJ, Dobbins CJ (1989) Comparing the short and long versions of the AIMS. J Rheumatol 16(8):1105

Zborowski M (1952) Cultural components in responses to pain. J Social Issues 8:16–30

Zola IK (1966) Culture and symptoms – an analysis of patients presenting complaints. Am Social Rev 31:615–630

The Assessment of Quality of Life in Refugees

J. De Vries and *G.L. Van Heck*

Summary

The millions of refugees in the world are a very vulnerable group. They are on the run from all kinds of violence. This obviously affects their physical and psychological health. Although these effects have been studied separately, the entire scope of problems is very rarely investigated. Even in Western countries, where quality of life (QOL) research is very common, the QOL of refugees has not been studied. However, mental health status has been a special subject of study in refugee camps. Those assessing QOL or its separate aspects encounter a number of problems like the use of adequate measures, translation equivalence, informed consent, and the fact that refugees, especially women, are reluctant to disclose their traumatic experiences. However, there are a number of ways to overcome these problems and they are outlined in the present chapter.

Introduction

Today we are facing a global refugee problem of unprecedented proportion. It is estimated that there are currently between 20 and 30 million refugees and displaced persons in the world (Jablensky et al. 1991). This number increases every day, due to civil wars in, for instance, Somalia and in the former Yugoslavia. In 1990, 15 million refugees were under the responsibility of the United Nations High Commissioner for Refugees (UNHCR). Most of these refugees only cross a border and thus do not seek asylum in a Western country. Six million eight hundred thousand of them live in Asia and 4600000 in Africa (De Jong 1991). As a consequence, refugees in Africa are being hosted by some of the poorest nations in the world (Harrell-Bond 1986). For example, in 1992 Malawi had more than one million Mozambican refugees (Ager 1992).

When a large group of refugees cross a border, the UNHCR establishes settlements. According to the 1951 Convention and the 1967 Protocol Relating to the Status of Refugees, refugees are persons who have left their countries of origin due to "a well-founded fear of being persecuted for reasons of race, religion, nationality, membership in a particular social group or political opinion."

J. Orley, W. Kuyken (Eds.)
Quality of Life Assessment:
International Perspectives

Governments in some parts of the world, for example most countries in Africa and the Central American countries, recognize persons to be refugees who are not necessarily the direct targets of persecution but have suffered violence, strife, war and similar politically generated disasters that affect whole groups rather than individuals. The overwhelming majority of the refugees under the UNHCR mandate are persons who meet the latter definition of refugees (Weiss Fagen 1990).

The Vulnerability of Refugees

Refugees are a very vulnerable group. This is not only because they suffered violence, war or persecution in their home country but also because, after their flight, they are commonly not protected by a government, and are often victims of violence. This is especially true for self-settled refugees. For instance, among the Ugandans who first went to Zaire and later to Sudan, 17% said they had come to a settlement because of harassment, while 28.5% of those who moved directly to the Sudan reported harassment as their reason for registering for settlement. In one study, unassisted refugees reported an overall average of 5.7 family members per household who had died during their flight from Uganda or in Sudan or Zaire. Also many family members were lost. There was a strong indication that experiences of death and violence accounted for the decisions of some households to give up independence and go to the settlements (Harrell-Bond 1986).

Furthermore, refugees are often not economically secure. For instance, Harrell-Bond (1986) pointed out that in Sudan healthy persons leave the refugee camp as soon as possible, leaving behind those who are vulnerable and thus decreasing the chances that the settlements could become viable agricultural economies. This situation was partly caused by the fact that people who moved to refugee camps were expected to make their living through agriculture, despite their background (e.g., high education or high-ranking jobs). When refugees arrived in a refugee camp, they were confronted with a loss of educational opportunities. Young people who had been going to school and were very keen to finish their education became listless, apathetic, angry, and sometimes even violent. In this context, Rangaraj (1988) cited the case of a young man who tried to commit suicide. Then, when this man was given books on electricity and an occupation he had practised years before he came to the refugee camp, his state of mind improved remarkably. Furthermore, Mollica et al. (1991) reported that, in their study in refugee camps in Thailand, one of four Khmer adults attended school and Khmer language and reading skills were the subjects most desired by the students.

Some other problems of refugees are grief, depression, anxiety, helplessness, and sleeplessness (e.g., Harrell-Bond 1986; Kroll et al. 1989; Lam and Westermeyer 1988; Mollica et al. 1991; Van Willigen 1993; Westermeyer 1989). These problems all constitute aspects of QOL.

Quality of Life of Refugees

In the last few decades, there has been an enormous amount of research on QOL. Providing the exact meaning of the term "QOL" is rather difficult, due to the fact that an elaborate theoretical framework is (still) lacking. Therefore, there are nearly as many definitions of QOL as there are studies on this subject (e.g., Andrews 1991; Badura and Waltz 1984; Campbell 1981; Karan et al. 1990).

In this chapter, QOL is defined as an individual's perception of his/her position in life in the context of the culture and value systems in which he/she lives and in relation to his/her goals, expectations, standards and concerns. It is a broad-ranging concept affected in a complex way by the person's physical health, psychological state, level of independence, social relationships, and relationship to salient features of his/her environment (WHOQOL Group 1993).

With a few exceptions, QOL is only a research subject in Western countries. Moreover, in studies on refugees the research is focussing only on separate aspects of QOL. For instance, in a study by Van Willigen (1993), refugees were found to report a number of physical complaints which were the result of strain, such as headache, fatigue, muscular pain, and joint pain. In this study, psychological complaints referred predominantly to trouble sleeping, feelings of anxiety, aggressive behaviour, concentration and memory disorders, nightmares, and depression. Lin et al. (1985) studied Chinese, Vietnamese, Lowland Laotian, and Mien refugees as well as immigrants from China and the Filipinos in primary care in the USA. They found that 25% of the reasons given to visit a clinic were ill-defined somatic symptoms such as headache, abdominal pain, low back pain, insomnia, and dizziness. For the Vietnamese, older age, being single, large household size, and lack of proficiency in English were associated with vague somatic symptoms in the absence of a detectable etiology.

Post-Traumatic Stress Disorder

Mollica et al. (1987) investigated psychiatric patients in the USA from Cambodian, Hmong, Laotian, and Vietnamese origin. They found that 50% suffered from post-traumatic stress disorder (PTSD), a syndrome of stress reactions to traumatic incidents. According to the ICD-10 (World Health Organization 1992), there are three groups of symptoms of PTSD: 1) re-experience phenomena; 2) avoidance and numbing phenomena; and 3) symptoms of increased arousal. Stress reactions to traumatic incidents can be understood essentially as the reactions of normal human beings to sudden, unexpected and terrifying events in their lives (Hodgkinson and Stewart 1991). Research done by Shinfuku (1993) in a refugee camp revealed that more than 85% of the Cambodian refugees suffered from PTSD occurring after an intensely traumatic event. It was shown that the effects could extend over a long period of time. In addition, various kinds of psychosomatic symptoms that are related to depression can coincide with PTSD. In a study on Southeast Asian refugees (Kroll et al. 1989) who were in contact with a community clinic in the USA, major depressive episode was the most common diagnosis. The percentage of subjects suffering from major depression ranged from 54.1% in Vietnamese refugees to 80.4% in Hmong. In Hmong, Laotian, and Cambodian refugees, PTSD was the second most established psychiatric diagnosis, followed by anxiety and somatoform disorders. In Vietnamese refugees, anxiety, somatoform disorders and schizophrenia formed the second most common diagnoses (10.8%), followed by PTSD. According to Westermeyer (1989), refugees have consistently shown some of the highest rates of psychopathology among all types of migrants.

Basic Physical Needs and Psychological Adaptation

In refugee camps the major focus is on basic physical needs of the masses. These basic physical aspects are nutrition, water and sanitation, and security. Malnutrition and starvation can lead to stunted growth, mental deficiency, and brain damage in infants, children, adolescents, and lactating mothers (Jablensky et al. 1991). In refugees, vitamin A deficiency is a serious public health problem. Each year some 250000 children are irreversibly blinded due to the effects on the eye of vitamin A shortage (xerophthalmia). This deficiency can occur at any age, but the most severe effects are usually found in pre-school children. In refugee populations, older children and adults may also be at risk (Refugee Participation Network 1992). Furthermore, it is widely recognized that, without the provision of clean water, a stable food supply, basic sanitation and the elimination of such environmental risks as the mosquito or the tsetse fly, very little "development", societal transformation or improvement in health care is likely to occur. In particular the food supply, quantitative as well as qualitative, is not only important to the physical health and survival of people, but also for the psychological adaptation of people. The effects of natural starvation generally tend to be severe and widely variable because there is not only calorie reduction but also exacerbating factors such as dietary deficiencies, and societal disruptions are generally present.

The characteristic set of behavioural changes which were observed in both the natural and experimental conditions included depression, irritability, nervousness, obliteration of sex drive, loss of concentration, apathy, loss of concern with the niceties, and an overriding concern with food and eating. Significantly, these behaviours do not quickly disappear after relief from food deprivation, but persist for several months even if an unlimited good diet is available. The shortage of nutritious food may itself be the basis for many of the psychosocial problems and the behaviours associated with the so-called "dependency syndrome."

"Dependency syndrome" is a term used for all undesirable social behaviour found in the settlements (Harrell-Bond 1986). For instance, Rangaraj (1988) reported abnormal forms of behaviour and instances of antisocial behaviour. Furthermore, Harrell-Bond (1986) reported neglect of environmental health among settlements in Sudan as one of the most serious symptoms of this so-called "dependency syndrome." In contrast, Mollica et al. (1991) found that all their respondents indicated high levels of personal hygiene despite scarce water resources. Jablensky et al. (1991), however, mentioned poor physical health – which is directly or indirectly linked to poor sanitation, poor nutrition, crowding, and the absence of basic shelter – as a risk factor in refugee status. Eighty-seven per cent of the adult Khmer respondents rated their own health status as "fair" to "poor" in a study by Mollica et al. (1991). This poor health status was associated with the presence of common medical conditions in the camp. On top of this, almost 10% of the respondents indicated suffering from a head injury or seizures.

Social and Psychological Problems

Although basic physical needs are important, attention should also be paid to other domains of QOL, namely the *social* and *psychological* problems of refugees. However, as mentioned above, QOL as such is not a topic in studies on refugees. This situation is shown by the fact that in "An Annotated Bibliography on Refugee Mental Health" (Williams 1987), as well as in "A Selected Bibliography on Refugee Health" (Thoolen and Forbes Martin, 1991), QOL was not an entry in the Subject Index. Moreover, there is only one reference on QOL and refugees in Psychlit (a version of Psychological Abstracts on CD rom). This reference was a study by Fazel and Young (1988) on life quality of Tibetans and Hindus. In this study the perceived QOL was measured with the Quality of Life scale, which consists of 17 items selected from the survey of Andrews and Withey (1976). The questions were translated from English to the appropriate languages. The Tibetans seemed to have a higher QOL than the Hindus. The difference between the QOL of the Hindus and the Tibetans was explained in terms of religion. The only other study on QOL and refugees known to us is one done by Ager (1992). He investigated the QOL among Mozambican refugees in Malawi. The emphasis in his concept of QOL was on the *objective* aspects, such as physiological needs like food and water, safety needs like clothing, and shelter. The other needs that he paid attention to were belonging needs, esteem needs, and transcendance needs. However, he did not ask people, for instance, whether they wanted to belong to a particular group of people. Instead, he asked a number of objective questions from which he deduced the extent of the belonging needs. Thus, the *perceived* quality of life of refugees has not yet been assessed.

By now it will be clear that, besides the basic physical needs, many other aspects of QOL are important to refugees, too. For instance, Harrell-Bond (1986) found that the demands of individual survival undermine social values, and the time that it takes for new supportive social units to establish themselves in the absence of kinsfolk is long. However, in a survey by Mollica et al. (1991), one-third of the respondents indicated they took care of someone who did not live with them, such as an elderly person and/or disabled or sick persons. This does point to a new supportive system. The essential disabilities suffered by refugees could be grouped under three categories: 1) their powerlessness vis-à-vis an alien social and economic environment. This has to do with the fact that refugees also need such basics as training in language, or information concerning soil conditions, rainfall patterns, or crop suitability which has often been overlooked. It is known that people often have culture shock when they move to another country (Westermeyer 1986). This situation can lead to psychological effects like sleepiness, apathy, depression, compulsive eating or drinking, homesickness, and exaggerated yearning for all things and friends of their own country, insecurity of professional judgement, negative stereotyping of illnesses, and obsession with cleanliness. Children may show regression in toilet training or social behaviour, interrupted sleep, skin eruptions, and stomach disorders. Older children may manifest difficulty in maintaining academic competence, working out their anxiety in disruptive behaviour and sometimes even experimenting with drugs, alcohol, and sex (Harrell-Bond, 1986); 2) the physical and psychological toll on individuals, which has immediate and long-term consequences for the capacity of the society to re-establish viable production units (e.g., Jablensky et al. 1991; Mollica et al. 1991; Rangaraj 1988; Westermeyer 1989); and 3) the loss of property, perhaps the most general characteristic of all refugees (Harrell-Bond 1986; Westermeyer 1989).

In southern Sudan, there was evidence which suggested that few refugees escaped the psychological scars of flight and exile (Harrell-Bond 1986). Refugees are regularly confronted with their traumas through recurrent thoughts and dreams (e.g., Mollica et al. 1991; Tek et al. 1992; Van Willigen 1993). Studies among survivors of concentration camps reported remarkably consistent symptoms, including chronic depression, anxiety, sleep disorders, fatigue, recurring nightmares, isolation, rumination, irritability, and a hyperactive startle reaction (Kinzie et al. 1984).

Psychological Stress and Negative Affect

There have been a number of studies on *psychological stress* among refugees. For instance, Harrell-Bond (1986) organised a drawing contest for refugee children in Sudan. The assignment was to draw impressions of refugee life. Judged by the drawings, the word refugee itself seemed to be associated in the minds of children with their experiences of violence, death, and starvation. A follow-up after one year yielded the same results. Moreover, the themes of songs composed by adults in exile showed a preoccupation with death, suffering, hunger, and violent revenge.

Psychological stress includes being tortured, observing the torture or murder of others, separation from loved ones, robbery, incarceration for one's political or religious beliefs or one's national identity, the wounding or death of friends and relatives, social upheaval, rejection by one's fellow citizens, the loss of one's home and occupation, inability to protect one's spouse or children, exposure to political terrorism, and uncertainty for the future. These experiences are often associated with PTSD (Westermeyer 1989) as well as with other psychological problems. For instance, Mollica et al. (1991) found in a study on Khmer adults that 83% suffered from depression. Also recurrent memory phenomena such as memories, nightmares, dreams, and the reliving of the traumatic events were common. Fifteen per cent of the respondents met the Western criteria of PTSD. Also 29% mentioned feeling extremely hopeless and ashamed. Other trauma-related symptoms were, for example, trouble sleeping (extreme: 17%), inability to remember (extreme: 15%), feeling guilty for having survived (extreme: 12%), and feeling that one has no future (extreme: 32%). The proportion of adults with poor health status (87%) was almost exactly equivalent to the proportion that claimed to have depression (83%). Twenty per cent indicated that they had severe to moderate bodily pain. The presence of pain was associated with poor health status, depression and the perception of health impairment of social functioning. In addition, respondents were asked to report the trauma experiences in the past year. Fifty-two per cent reported lack of food or water, 6% had had a lack of shelter, and 5% had had a serious injury. However, a lot of respondents had witnessed traumatic experiences. For example, 24% of the respondents reported having been a witness to a serious injury; 20% had witnessed an imprisonment. Depression and hopelessness were highly associated with trauma-related symptoms.

Survival guilt is very common in survivors of disasters (Hodgkinson and Stewart 1991). Tobin and Friedman (1983) reported survival guilt as well as Oriental nightmare deaths in refugees. These deaths presumably occurred as a result of a nightmare in which a big person sits on the dreamer until he or she chokes.

Tek et al. (1992) reported that torture victims showed a number of somatic and psychological symptoms. The most common somatic symptom was pain. The psychological symptoms associated with torture were sleeping disorders, fatigue, impaired concentration, nightmares, low tolerance, anxiety, impaired memory, depression, sexual problems, reduced ability and desire for contact, and panic attacks. According to Bamber (1988), the rationale for torture was that isolation, humiliation, psychological pressure, and physical pain are means to obtain information, to break down the prisoner, and to intimidate those close to him or her.

In Sudan, a study was done among adult refugees in a settlement, both self-settled refugees and Sudanese. The total number of subjects was 57. The results were that 13 persons were diagnosed as having no psychiatric problems; 17 persons were suffering anxiety; 6 persons were suffering anxiety with depressive features; 19 persons suffered from depression; and 11 persons suffered from depression with anxiety features. The depressives presented primarily somatic symptoms such as headaches, bodies which ached even when they did no work, constant exhaustion, anergy and retardation, sleeplessness, loss of appetite, and loss of libido (Harrell-Bond 1986). Rangaraj (1988) also found mainly somatic complaints. However, he also reported that 60% of the symptoms could be classified under anxiety and depression.

All Khmer consider themselves victims of violence because they either witnessed violence or underwent it themselves. For instance, the Cambodians who fled to Thailand were often attacked by pirates who raped the women. Husbands and fiancés who had witnessed the raping of their wives or fiancées suffered from their failure to protect the women. They avoided talking to each other about the trauma suffered. However, usually the husband or fiancé projected his feeling of guilt onto someone else. The husband or fiancé who did not project his guilt onto his wife or fiancée, or onto someone else, could suffer from depression, which began by devaluing himself (Khuong 1988). Khmer respondents revealed extensive use of avoidance behaviour to help them escape the emotional upset of their traumatic life experiences. This was considered a positive coping strategy (Mollica et al. 1991). Extremely stressful situations, social isolation, depression, alcohol and drug abuse, organic brain impairment, and paranoid reactions can activate violence in refugee families (Lam and Nguyen 1988). Anger, aggression, violent behaviour, and drug and alcohol abuse were also mentioned by Jablensky et al. (1991) as manifestations of psychosocial maladjustment.

In a study by Harrell-Bond (1986), marital status – where spouses were present – appeared positively related to mental health. Similarly the presence of an individual's close relatives other than the spouse seemed negatively related with suffering depression. Kroll et al. (1989), in a study on Southeast Asian refugees living in the USA, found that women who were widows had significantly more depressive and anxiety symptoms than women who were not widows. In the survey by Mollica et al. (1991), PTSD was more common in widows. An earlier study by Mollica et al. (1987) made the striking finding that Cambodian women who did not have spouses had experienced more traumatic experiences than all other clinical subgroups.

Adverse life events are a cause of depression, though there are complex factors which make some people more vulnerable to them than others. Refugees in Africa have not only experienced the loss of roots, geography, emotional support, and the culture and status they enjoyed before flight; the scale of death from military violence, illness, and malnutrition is great (Harrell-Bond 1986). In 1989 Westermeyer also noted a number of losses that refugees incurred, including loss of country, home, work, social order, and social network, and often loss of family, friends, relatives and health. The loss of a country and, in addition, often the loss of at least one close relative are characteristic for all refugees.

Shinfuku (1993) found that the impact of traumatic events on people and the degree of PTSD are related to the number and severity of the traumatic events experienced. For instance, Carlson and Rosser-Hogan (1991) found in a group of Cambodian refugees a relationship between the amount of trauma experienced and PTSD and the number of traumatic events and the severity of psychiatric symptoms such as dissociation, depression, and anxiety. Research with Khmer adults also revealed that PTSD is positively associated with the number of traumatic events experienced (Mollica et al. 1987, 1991). In the 1987 study, patients with the diagnosis of PTSD reported twice as many traumatic events compared with patients having other psychiatric diagnoses. Another identified close link was between depression and the scale of an individual's losses (Harrell-Bond 1986).

Grief

Due to their losses, many refugees experience *grief.* Grief can itself cause temporary psychological dislocation and great distress in everyone. It is a universal reaction to bereavement. The main components of grief are: 1) shock. In this stage it is as if feelings have been turned off; 2) disorganisation characterised by confusion, poor concentration, and memory lapses; 3) denial of the facts or meaning of the loss; 4) depression; 5) guilt; 6) anxiety; 7) aggression; 8) resolution and acceptance; and 9) reintegration (Hodgkinson and Stewart 1991). Lam and Westermeyer (1988) stated that sleep disturbance, appetite disturbance, absent-mindedness, social withdrawal, dreaming, treasuring objects, avoiding objects, crying, and depression are all possible behavioural reactions of grief. They further mentioned feelings of sadness, anger, guilt, anxiety, loneliness, shock and helplessness, emancipation, relief, and numbness. Finally, they mentioned four accompanying thought patterns; *viz,* disbelief, confusion, sense of presence, and illusions.

Grief work demands time, energy, and a degree of security which the victim may not possess in the midst of dealing with harsh realities. Prolonged residence in refugee camps and other types of relocation camps over months or years can create a state of resentful apathy and dependence (Westermeyer 1989).

From the above, it is clear that the traumas related to (the cause of) the flight and the subsequent new living conditions affect all aspects of QOL of refugees. Therefore, the physical, social and psychological aspects should not be studied separately but all at the same time. However, the assessment of QOL in refugees is related to a number of methodological problems.

Difficulties in Assessing QOL in Refugees: Practical and Methodological Obstacles

Environmental Diversity

The first problem stems from the fact that there are many different types of refugee camps. For instance, some camps are typical starting camps. As a consequence, life in this living environment is rather chaotic and usually unsafe. Undoubtedly, such a camp is rather distinct from a more or less settled camp that offers some stability and security. Furthermore, camps not only differ in terms of the amount of orderliness and regulation or the amount of shelter that they can offer but also vary in terms of their temporal aspects. It really matters whether or not a particular camp is a rather permanent place or is meant to be closed within a short period of time, implying the resettlement of refugees back home or to another camp.

Assessment of QOL should take into account these different "characteristics" of the environment. This requires a thorough study of the ecological context of behaviour, including both the social and physical components of everyday settings for goal-directed, purposive behaviour (e.g., Harrell-Bond 1986; Jablensky et al. 1991). What should be scrutinized are the "affordances" of the environment (cf. Gibson 1979), that is, what the camp environment offers, provides, or furnishes.

In this context, studies of the behaviour settings within a camp (cf. Barker 1968) can provide a useful tool for situational analysis. The essential properties of a behavioural setting are as follows: 1) standing extra-individual patterns of behaviour with specific temporal-spatial coordinates; 2) constellations of non-behavioural (physical, geographical) setting elements; 3) the fact that the physical-geographical-temporal environment is circumjacent to and synomorphic with the standing patterns of behaviour, and 4) the interdependence within a given behaviour setting of the various configurations of physical and behavioural attributes (see also Schoggen 1989). The study of behaviour settings can help to maintain the QOL in isolated communities (Bechtel 1982) and to analyse adaptation to environmental change.

A somewhat related approach may be based on the insider perceptions of human environments (cf. Moos 1973). A good example of this is the work of Pace and Stern (1958; Stern 1970). Using Murray's (1938) views on personal needs and environmental presses, Pace and Stern (1958) found that the "personalities" of environments could be described in ways paralleling the personalities of people. Unlike Barker's approach, the work of Pace and Stern introduces perceived presses in the description of the environment; consistent with the Barker tradition, the assessment focuses on very concrete instances.

Instability of Camp Population

As mentioned above, it often happens that persons with the highest adaptative resources leave the refugee camp at their earliest convenience, whereas the people who lack these characteristics have to stay in the camp (see Harrell-Bond 1986). This situation has profound effects on the QOL of the camp community. When assessing the refugee QOL, this process of moving and transition – with the inevitable outcome that the most vulnerable are left behind – should be taken into account, because the availability of social support and of models for identification and learning can change drastically as a function of the exodus of the persons who are best suited for camp life.

Ways of Collecting Data

Assessors will be confronted rather often with the impossibility of using particular modes of data collection (Van de Vijver and Poortinga 1991). First, there is the problem of illiteracy. This blocks the use of traditional paper-and-pencil tests and more or less forces the use of structured or semi-structured interviews (Berry et al. 1992). In certain respects, interviews are superior to questionnaires because they offer the opportunity to scrutinize some topics in more detail, not being restricted by the prescribed set of questionnaire items. The other side of the coin is, of course, that semi-structured and unstructured interviews form a less standardized procedure. Another relevant point here concerns the fact that interviews never can provide the perceived safety of the anonymous condition inherent in questionnaire use.

Another problem investigators have to face is the language problem which makes it necessary to work with bilingual workers. In the process of translation, discrepancies can occur between the original answers and the translated versions, due either to attempts to control deliberately the information which proceeds between refugee and professional, or without any intention of doing so (Hunt et al. 1991; Van de Vijver and Poortinga 1991; Westermeyer 1986). Thus a bilingual worker can convey the refugee's thoughts and feelings to the professional in an accurate fashion but still not convey the full clinical import of these messages to the professional. According to Westermeyer (1986), the critical elements in the translator/interpreter-professional relationship are: 1) mutual understanding, 2) trust, 3) experience in working together, and 4) some routine for who does what, when, and how. Naturally this relationship requires some time to develop. In Westermeyer's (1986, p. 27) words: "Expecting bilinguals and professionals to work together without a period of mutual orientation and teamwork experience (as is often done by refugee program directors) is unrealistic." We fully agree with Westermeyer that there is urgent need for training of bilingual workers. Such training should not focus exclusively on denotative and connotative translation, interpretation and negotiation, but should also be directed at the study of the basic principles of biopsychosocial approaches to health and well-being (see Westermeyer 1986, for a detailed list of desiderata and criteria).

Then, there is the problem of measuring QOL in people who are less able or unable to speak for themselves, *viz*, children and persons with some type of handicap, for instance deaf individuals or persons with mental retardation (see e.g., Taylor and Bogdan 1990). Especially for young children, self-reports cannot be obtained and consequently one has to rely upon answers provided by proxies.

Self-Disclosure: Reluctance to Cooperate

Self-disclosure has a beneficial effect upon well-being (Pennebaker et al. 1988). According to De Jong (1991, p. 5), "Disclosing traumatic experiences is psychologically and physically beneficial. Inhibition of trauma-related thoughts or feelings requires physiological work that serves as a cumulative stressor over time." In spite of this, in refugees one has to expect a great reluctance to disclose themselves.

There are several reasons for this state of affairs. First, people can be so seriously traumatized that they feel unable to report on their present state. Second, a refusal to cooperate can be based upon a profound lack of trust, sometimes even resulting in some paranoid state. Third, in some cultures people are not inclined to talk about their traumatic experiences. For example, Khmer adults are inclined to conceive of avoidance as a highly adequate coping mechanism (Mollica et al. 1991). The respondents also revealed that an extensive use of avoidance behaviour was effective in helping them to overcome the emotional distress resulting from their traumatic life experiences. Finally, refugee women with a history of sexual violence rarely directly provide information about sexual violence to interviewers. It should be remembered that, in certain cultures, sexuality is a taboo issue and raped women are considered to be a shame to their families (Bredero 1984; De Neef and De Ruiter 1984). As a consequence, the history of rape trauma is usually revealed through veiled accounts of personal trauma in comments from family members (Mollica et al. 1987).

In a recent study, Mollica and co-workers (1992), demonstrated that, under favourable conditions in which confidentiality, informed consent, and respect for the patient are obvious, refugees have less difficulty telling their trauma history.

Available Instruments

There is a lack of properly restandardized questionnaires for use in populations of refugees in non-Western countries. Often only mechanical translations of Western instruments are used. In a few cases, however, carefully constructed instruments are used, the end-result of a construction process featuring the use of expert panels, proper back-translations, and methods for resolving differences. A rather good example of a scale that was constructed following adequate procedures is the Harvard Trauma Questionnaire (Mollica et al. 1992).

Unfortunately, most of the time scales that are employed in refugee studies do not meet high standards of psychometric quality. Frequently, instruments are used that are not equivalent to the original measures. For instance, many scales are not comparable in regards to style and connotation. A related shortcoming concerns the fact that many tests disregard the existence of culture-specific symptoms.

Recommendations

There are a number of ways to tackle the assessment problems mentioned above. Concerning the different types of refugee camps, for instance, in order to obtain full cooperation one has to stress the scientific and practical importance of a study for respondents as well as camp officers. This will be especially necessary when one wants to study a new, chaotic and unsafe camp. With respect to reliability of measures, it should be realised that it will always remain difficult to obtain test-retest scores or to assess QOL *in time*, when the population of a camp is unstable.

The consent of respondents has a very positive effect on honesty and openness. A confidential atmosphere can be a further factor in the stimulation of respondents. In this respect, the cultural background and gender of the interviewer will probably be of great influence. It is known that respondents are more open to an interviewer of the same cultural background, language, and gender. Gender might be very vital in getting information, especially from refugee women, concerning traumatic experiences like rape.

The interviews should be structured or at least semi-structured and the interviewers should be trained to receive standardised information. However, this will not eliminate the disadvantages completely.

A solution to the issue of translation is the development of a method by which one works with monolinguals as well as bilinguals (cf. Hunt et al. 1991). This is important because bilinguals usually have a higher educational level than most respondents. Therefore, it is possible that a translation will not be understandable to everyone. A monolingual with a lower educational level can check the text for comprehensibility.

Apart from the reliability and validity issues, an instrument that claims to measure QOL in refugees should be developed within the particular culture, using the target language. To get a subjective point of view, one can use the focus group methodology. Furthermore, an instrument that is used to measure QOL in refugee camps preferably should be constructed on the spot, taking into account the existence of culture-specific symptoms. Inherent in refugee research is the fact that one has to work under very difficult circumstances, requiring an ability to adapt to interruptions and to improvise in unexpected situations. However, this does not mean that one is absolved from the obligation of working with the best possible measures.

References

Ager A (1992) Quality of life amongst Mozambican refugees in Malawi. A report to the Division of Mental Health, WHO, Geneva

Andrews FM (1991) Stability and change in levels and structure of subjective well-being: USA 1972 and 1988. Social Indicators Res 25:1–30

Andrews FM, Withey SB (1976) Social indicaters of well-being: Americans' perceptions of life quality. Plenum Press, New York

Badura B, Waltz M (1984) Social support and the quality of life following myocardial infarction. Social Indicators Res 14:295–311

Bamber H (1988) Torture and the infliction of other forms or organized violence. In: Miserez D (ed) Refugees – the trauma of exile: the humanitarian role of Red Cross and Red Crescent. Martinus Nijhoff Publishers, Dordrecht, pp 45–53

Barker RG (1968) Ecological psychology: concepts and methods for studying the environment of human behaviour. Palo Alto, CA, Stanford University Press

Bechtel RB (1982) Contributions of ecological psychology to the evaluation of environments. Internat Rev Appl Psychol 31:153–167

Berry JW, Poortinga YH, Segall MH, Dasen PR (1992) Cross-cultural psychology: research and applications. Cambridge University Press, New York

Bredero M (1984) Anna en al die duizenden anderen [Anna and all those thousands of other women]. Opzij 12:16–18
Campbell A (1981) The sense of well-being in America. McGraw-Hill, New York
Carlson EB, Rosser-Hogan R (1991) Trauma experiences, posttraumatic stress, dissociation, and depression in Cambodian refugees. Am J Psychiat 148:1548–1551
De Jong JTVM (1991) IPSER-WHO-WFMII program on the identification, management and prevention of psychosocial and mental health problems of refugees and victims of man-made disaster within primary health care. IPSER, Maastricht
De Neef CEJ, De Ruiter SJ (1984) Seksueel geweld tegen vrouwelijke vluchtelingen: rapport over de aard en gevolgen van seksueel geweld dat deze vrouwen elders hebben ondergaan [Sexual violence against female refugees: report on the nature and consequences of sexual violence that these women have undergone elsewhere]. Ministerie van Sociale Zaken en Werkgelegenheid, Den Haag
Fazel MK, Young DM (1988) Life Quality of Tibetans and Hindus: a function of religion. Scientific Study Religion 27:229–242
Gibson JJ (1979) The ecological approach to visual perception. Houghton Mifflin, Boston
Harrell-Bond BE (1986) Imposing aid: emergency assistance to refugees. Oxford University Press, New York
Hodgkinson PE, Stewart M (1991) Coping with catastrophe: a handbook of disaster management. Routledge, London
Hunt SM, Alonso J, Bucquet D, Niero M, Wiklund I, McKenna S (1991) Cross-cultural adaptation of health measures. Health Pol 19:33–44
Jablensky A, Marsella AJ, Ekblad S, Jansson B, Levi L (1991) Stress research reports. The First International Conference on the Mental Health and Wellbeing of the World's Refugees and Displaced Persons. Stockholm
Karan OC, Lambour G, Greenspan S (1990) Persons in transition. In: Schalock RL (ed) Quality of life: perspectives and issues. American Association on Mental Retardation, Washington, pp 85–92
Khuong DT (1988) Victims of violence in the South China Sea. In: Miserez D (ed) Refugees – the trauma of exile: the humanitarian role of the Red Cross and the Red Crescent. Martinus Nijhoff Publishers, Dordrecht, pp 18–38
Kinzie JD, Fredrickson RH, Ben R, Fleck J, Karls W (1984) Posttraumatic stress disorder among survivors of Cambodian concentration camps. Am J Psychiat 141:645–650
Kroll J, Habenicht M, Mackenzie MD, Yang M, Chan S, Vang T, Nguyen T, Ly M, Phommasouvanh R, Nguyen H, Vang Y, Souvannasoth L, Cabugao R (1989) Depression and posttraumatic stress disorder in Southeast Asian refugees. Am J Psychiat 146: 1592–1597
Lam L, Nguyen H (1988) Domestic violence in refugee families. Refugee Mental Health Lett 2:5–9
Lam L, Westermeyer J (1988) Grief reactions in the refugee. Refugee Mental Health Lett 2:2–9
Lin EHB, Carter WB, Kleinman AM (1985) An exploration of somatization among Asian refugees and immigrants in primary care. Am J Public Health 75:1080–1084
Mollica RF, Wyshak G, Lavelle J (1987) The psychosocial impact of war trauma and torture on Southeast Asian refugees. Am J Psychiat 144:1567–1572
Mollica RF, Donelan K, Svang Tor BA, Lavelle J, Blaas C, Frankel M, Bennett D, Blendon RJ (1991) Repatriation and disability: a community study of health, mental health, and social functioning of the Khmer residents of Site Two. World Federation for Mental Health, unpublished report
Mollica RF, Caspi-Yavin Y, Bollini P, Truong T, Tor S, Lavelle J (1992) The Harvard Trauma Questionnaire: Validating a cross-cultural instrument for measuring torture, trauma, and post-traumatic stress disorder in Indochinese refugees. J Nervous Mental Dis 180: 111–116
Moos RH (1973) Conceptualization of human environments. Am Psychol 32:246–254
Murray HA (1938) Explorations in personality. New York, Oxford University Press

Pace CR, Stern GG (1958) An approach to the measurement of psychological characteristics of college environments. J Educ Psychol 49:269–277
Pennebaker JW, Kiecolt-Glaser JK, Glaser R (1988) Disclosure of trauma and immune function: Health implications for psychotherapy. J Consulting Clin Psychol 56:239–245
Rangaraj AG (1988) The health status of refugees in South East Asia. In: Miserez D (ed) Refugees – the trauma of exile: the humanitarian role of Red Cross and Red Crescent. Martinus Nijhoff Publishers, Dordrecht, pp 39–44
Refugee Participation Network (1992) Vitamin A deficiency and the eye. Refugee Participation Network 12:21–22
Schoggen P (1989) Behaviour settings. A revision and extension of Roger G. Barker's ecological psychology. Stanford University Press, Stanford, CA
Shinfuku N (1993) Mission report on the mental health programme in Cambodia. Unpublished report, WHO
Stern GG (1970) People in context: measuring person-environment congruence in education and industry. Wiley, New York
Taylor SJ, Bogdan R (1990) Quality of life and the individual's perspective. In: Schalock RL (ed) Quality of life: perspectives and issues. Association on Mental Retardation, Washington, pp 27–40
Tec C et al (1992) The Ankara experience: torture is no stranger to the soil of Asia Minor – almost an old friend. Torture 2:41–42
Thoolen H, Forbes Martin S (1991) A selected bibliography on refugee health. UNHCR, Geneva
Tobin JJ, Friedman J (1983) Spirits, shamans, and nightmare death: survivor stress in a Hmong refugee. Am J Orthopsychiat 53:439–448
Van de Vijver FJR, Poortinga YH (1991) Testing across cultures. In: Hambleton RK, Zaal IN (eds) Advances in educational and psychological testing: Theory and applications. Kluwer Academic Publishers, Boston/London/Dordrecht
Van Willigen L (1993) Psychische problemen door uitzichtloosheid onder vluchtelingen. Het Nieuwsblad June 5, 31
Weiss Fagen P (1990) Worldwide refugees: problem of disruption, fear, and poverty. In: Holtzman WH, Bornemann TH (eds) Mental health of immigrants and refugees. Hogg Foundation for Mental Health, Austin, pp 7–15
Westermeyer J (1986) Models of assessment, treatment, and prevention for social adjustment and mental health of refugees. Unpublished Report, University of Minnesota
Westermeyer J (1989) Mental health for refugees and other migrants: social and preventive approaches. Charles C Thomas, Springfield, IL
WHO (1992) The ICD-10 classification of mental and behavioural disorders: clinical descriptions and diagnostic guidelines. WHO, Geneva
WHOQOL Group (1993) Study protocol for the World Health Organization project to develop a quality of life assessment instrument (WHOQOL). Quality Life Res 2:153–159
Williams CL (1987) An annotated bibliography on refugee mental health. DHSS Publication, Washington, DC

Quality of Life in Hypertensives and Normotensives in Israel: Introducing a Self-Structured Subjective Measure

M. Amir, D. Bar-on and *N. Cristal*

Summary

The objective of the present report was to introduce and evaluate a new, qualitative, self-structured measure of quality of life (QOL) as part of a battery of instruments measuring this concept. The study compared the pre- and post-treatment evaluation of 268 men between the ages of 40 and 65 with mild hypertension, randomly allocated to one of three treatment groups in a double-blind design, with evaluations of 155 normotensive subjects who were matched for age and level of education. The groups were treated with two antihypertensive drugs, Isradipine and Methyldopa, in addition to a placebo.

We found that the new measure showed both internal reliability and construct validity. When spouses and physicians were asked about the patients' QOL, we found that they were only in moderate agreement with the patients' own definition of their QOL.

We found that the normotensives have better QOL than the hypertensives on most pre-structured measures. They also view health issues as less important than the hypertensive patients. Both groups view family values as the most important aspect of their QOL. It is suggested that this result might be idiosyncratic to a Jewish society, where family values are considered of great importance; further cross-cultural research will answer whether this is true for other societies as well.

Introduction

QOL in hypertension has become an important issue in recent years. The disease is thought to have few symptoms, in contrast to certain pharmacological treatments which have been reported to produce adverse reactions, such as sleep, sex and memory disorders (Testa et al. 1993). Furthermore, it is not clear what the concept of QOL includes and how it is assessed in this particular disease, in which the relationship between mind, body and soul is poorly understood. A review of 240 articles appearing in medical journals between 1977 to 1990 that referred to the QOL of hypertensives showed that there were only 26 studies that had obtained the necessary and sufficient statistical data to be included in a detailed meta-analysis (Bar-on and Yaniv, manuscript in preparation). This meta-analysis concluded that the overall effect on the QOL

J. Orley, W. Kuyken (Eds.)
Quality of Life Assessment:
International Perspectives

was insignificant. The studies included in the meta-analysis were all conducted between 1985 and 1990, suggesting that little or no progress has taken place in the measurement of QOL during these years. These studies, reflecting the majority of studies in the field of QOL, all used pre-structured, quantitative measures of QOL (Croog et al. 1986; Siegriest et al. 1987; Testa et al. 1991).

Golombiewski et al. (1976) found that some subjects do not attach the same meaning to the pre-structured scales at repeated measurements; therefore, to understand changes in QOL one has to correct for this subjective cognitive bias.

These considerations led us to the following conceptual and methodological questions:

1) Who should determine what constitutes the patients' QOL: the patient, the physician, the spouse or the researcher? Do the pre-structured, quantitative measures give us adequate information about the patients' perception of his QOL?
2) What are the differences between QOL among hypertensives and normotensives before the influence of pharmacological treatment?
3) What are the influences on QOL of hypertensives in a clinical trial of two antihypertensive drugs, Methyldopa and Isradipine.

To test these questions we developed a qualitative self-structured measure of QOL which inquired into the subjective perception of hypertensives and normotensives as to the domains comprising their QOL. This measure, as well as pre-structured, formerly tested instruments, was given to patients undergoing the clinical trial and to a control group of normotensives.

Subjects and Methods

Subjects. A total of 368 male patients, 40–65 years old, with mild hypertension were randomly placed into three treatment groups – Methyldopa, Isradipine and placebo – in a double-blind design. After discontinuation and dropouts, 268 patients were available for comparison with 155 normotensive subjects, who were matched for age and education. (For a detailed description of the design of this study, see Yodfat and Cristal 1993).

QOL assessment. The hypertensives were interviewed at three times: before entry into the study, at 6 months, and at the end of the trial, at 12 months. Physicians provided their estimates at all three times; spouses gave theirs at the beginning and end of the trial. Hypertensives were recruited from nine local Sick Fund clinics representing all major geographical regions in Israel. The normotensives were drawn from kibbutz settlements, local Sick Fund clinics and industrial plants.

Instruments. The QOL data were divided into two parts: a semi-structured interview and a self-report questionnaire. The interview included the new subjective measurement of QOL, life events and a semantic memory test. The questionnaire included questions about physical, sleep and sexual dysfunction, depression, hardiness and stress at the workplace (see below). The instruments used are described below:

Subjective Domains of Quality of Life

This scale was especially developed for the present study by Prof. Dan Bar-on, and is based on the idea that QOL is a highly subjective concept. The subject created his own QOL scale (Bar-on and Amir 1993), using the corrective evaluation following Golembiewski et al. (1976). The subject assessed three domains which constituted for him the most important aspects of his QOL. For each domain the subject was asked to define the qualitative optimal, current and dysfunctional levels. Next the subject was asked to evaluate the current functioning of the domains of his QOL on a scale from 1 to 6. For instance, if the subject said that the most important domain for him was the education of his children, the optimal level could be that they all got a university education; the dysfunctional level could be that one or more would drop out of high school. The current functioning could be that two of three children received a high school certificate and one continued to a higher education, a situation which the subject evaluated as 4 on the 6-point scale.

Israel PERI Life Event Scale

This scale is an adaptation of the Holmes and Rahe "Social Readjustment Rating Scale" (Holmes and Rahe 1967). In the present study two facets were added, "desirability" and "controllability", following Rhodewalt and Augustdottir (1986). Subjects reported both recent (RLE) and past (PLE) critical life events.

Semantic Memory

Following Weingartner et al. (1983), an experimental laboratory method was used to measure this higher mental function. The subjects were asked to name as many vegetables as possible within a time limit of 60 seconds, and, within another 60 seconds, as many musical instruments as possible.

Physical, Sleep and Sexual Dysfunctioning

Jenkin's questionnaire (Croog et al. 1986), consisting of 11 items, was used. The subject rated each item according to the number of days in the past month the dysfunctioning was observed. In addition, the subject was asked how many hours he slept at night, the frequency of sexual relations and intensity of physical activity.

Depression

Lubin's mood scale (Lubin and Himmelstein 1976) was used as a measure of depression. The subject was presented with 34 adjectives relating to his mood and general feelings and was asked to assess what was suitable for him.

Hardiness

Kobasa's original 50-item questionnaire (1979) was used.

Stress at Workplace

Frankenhauser's 13-item questionnaire (Frankenhauser and Gardell 1976) asked the subject to assess various stressful aspects at the workplace.

Results

The present analysis focuses on the initial and final evaluations and the difference between them. Although mid-year measurements on the QOL scales were obtained, these measurements turned out to conform with the final evaluation, except that the results were less significant.

Initially we measured the reliability and validity of all pre-structured components. A factor analysis was performed separately on each questionnaire at the initial and final evaluation. The identical and discrete factors were tested for internal reliability by Cronbach's alpha-test. The reliability scores mostly replicated the original questionnaires' reliability test. The next step was to test the validity of the new, self-structured QOL measure. This was done for the initial and final evaluation in terms of the quantitative ratings of the current level of the subjects' major QOL domain compared to the pre-structured measures. Results were further controlled for age and level of education. Table 1 shows

Table 1. Patients' initial and final QOL ratings of current level of major domain intercorrelated with other QOL measures

	Initial QOL (n = 324)	Final QOL (n = 246)
Age	NS	0.13*
Level of education	0.28**	0.22**
Physical dysfunction	−0.22**	−0.32**
Sexual dysfunction	−0.25**	−0.19**
Sleep dysfunction	−0.20*	−0.13*
Hardiness	0.20*	0.24**
Depression	−0.51**	−0.42**

Pearson correlations, NS, nonsignificant; *$p<0.05$; **$p<0.001$.

the patients' initial QOL ratings of current level of major domain intercorrelated with other QOL measures.

This table shows that the new measure had systematic construct validity in addition to the reliability seen in the similarity of the mid-year measures to the final ratings.

Qualitative and quantitative analyses of the self-structured QOL measure were done separately. The *qualitative* content analysis showed that subjects have a different view of QOL than that of either researchers of physicians. The majority of normotensives (59%) and hypertensives (64%) identified family issues as their major concern in the base line interview, and 91% of these repeated this definition in the post-treatment interview. Among family issues, relationships with children (36%) and spouses (18%) were the main issues. Among all subjects, 28% related to the major domain positively, whereas 45% cited problems, indicating a negative evaluation. The remainder referred to this domain in a mixed statement. Thirty-one percent of the subjects indicated internal control regarding the major QOL domain; 36% indicated external control (for instance, fate, luck and other people). The remainder indicated a mixed source of control. Whereas normotensive subjects cited work and social issues (25%) as being significantly more important than health issues (7%), the hypertensives cited more health issues (19%) than work and social issues (13%). The hypertensives also viewed their health issues significantly more negatively and as being less controllable than did the normotensive subjects. Table 2 shows the results of the content analysis of the subjective domains of QOL of hypertensives and normotensives at the initial measurement. The results in the post-treatment evaluation were similar.

In the *quantitative* analysis of the self-structured measure, the current level of the major domain was evaluated on a 6-point scale (1 being most desirable and 6 being least desirable). No significant differences were found in the pretreatment assessment among the randomized groups and normotensives. However, at the end of the year there were significant differences. The Isradipine group improved more than the other two randomized groups ($p<0.05$). Subjects were further questioned during the post-treatment interview as to changes that had happened during the study period (from 1 being much worse, 5 being

Table 2. Qualitative content analysis of subjective domains of QOL of hypertensives and normotensives at the initial measurement (percentages)

	Domain			
	Family	Health	Work	Social
Hypertensives (n = 195)	64	19	9	4
Normotensives (n = 155)	59	8	13	12

The Chi-square analysis of the difference between the groups was significant, $p<0.005$.

Table 3. Intercorrelations between patients' and spouses' QOL ratings (Pearson correlation, n = 61)

	Spouses	
	Initial	Final
Patients		
Initial	0.48**	0.39*
Final	0.29*	0.56**

*p<0.05; **p<0.56**

Table 4. Pearson correlation between patients' final QOL ratings and their physicians' ratings regarding physical, work, sleep, sexual and mental dysfunctioning (n = 239)

Physicians' dysfunction ratings[a]	Patients' ratings of QOL[b]	Level of education	Dysfunctions			Depression
			Physical	Sexual	Sleep	
Physical	−0.19*	−0.31**	0.28**	0.25**	0.18*	0.32**
Work	−0.16*	−0.31**	0.26**	0.17*	0.18*	0.30**
Sleep	−0.19*	NS	0.21**	NS	0.25**	0.22**
Sexual	−0.21**	NS	0.23**	0.22**	NS	0.13*
Mental	−0.19	NS	0.32**	0.14*	NS	0.30**

[a] The higher the physicians' dysfunction ratings, the worse the evaluation of their patients' condition on this domain
[b] The higher the rating of the QOL current level of the main domain, the closer it is to the optimal level
*p<0.05; **p<0.001; NS, nonsignificant.

the same, and 9 being much better). Among the randomized groups, the placebo group re-evaluated their major QOL domain as getting worse, compared to the Isradipine group who evaluated their QOL as improving and the Methyldopa group who did not observe any changes.

Regarding the question as to who should evaluate patients' QOL, we correlated spouses' and patients' QOL ratings. The results can be seen in Table 3.

Table 3 shows that patients and their spouses are in fairly good agreement about what comprises the patients' QOL. However, considering that the highest correlation, 0.56, still leaves 69% of the variance unexplained, they are still far from being close to fully agreeing on how the patient sees his QOL. Correlations between the physicians' perception of the patients' QOL and their own are, as expected, lower than those of the spouses, as can be seen from Table 4.

This table indicates that the physicians' ideas about their patients' QOL differ from those of the patients.

Next we compared the hypertensives and normotensives on our QOL measures. T-tests were performed between the means of the two groups and the results showed that the normotensives were better off on most measures; they see their life events – both recent and past – as more desirable ($p < 0.05$). They have higher semantic memory scores on both our measures. They have a better sex life ($p < 0.001$), feel more fit ($p < 0.001$), and feel more in control at their workplace ($p < 0.001$). They feel they have more strength ($p < 0.001$), less tension at work (0.001), and are hardier ($p < 0.001$) and less depressed ($p < 0.001$) than their hypertensive counterparts. No difference was found between the groups on the current level of functioning of the main domain on the subjective measure. As to life events, only past life events are seen as more severe among the hypertensives. These differences between the hypertensives and normotensives were apparent both before and after the clinical trial. The pharmacological treatment changed the QOL measures very little. Only two measures were significantly different at the post-treatment assessment; the Isradipine group and the placebo group showed a significant improvement in semantic memory.

Discussion

We have examined a new subjective measure for measuring QOL and compared it with pre-structured measures as well as with the evaluations of physicians and spouses. Our results suggest that our new measure shows both internal reliability and construct validity. The new measure shows new qualitative aspects of QOL that had not become apparent from earlier studies, i.e., the importance of family values, especially concerning children. Family functioning is usually not part of the battery of QOL measurements (Bar-on and Amir 1993; Croog et al. 1986; Smoller-Wasserheil et al. 1991) and, therefore, it is possible that our standard instruments do not cover the important aspects of QOL from the patients' perspective. We can ask whether this finding is specifically true in Israel, as family values are considered very central in the Jewish tradition, or whether the traditional QOL measurements are missing something very important cross-culturally. Further research, especially across cultures, is needed to answer this question.

We also showed the new measure to be sensitive to changes not being detected by the pre-structured measurements. The Isradipine group showed an improvement in this measure, whereas the pre-structured measures were not able to detect differences, with the exception of memory. It is suggested that our new measure, being subjective and self-structured, has a sensitivity not found through the standard instruments in the field of QOL research.

As to who should be asked about the QOL of the patient, our results clearly show that both spouses and physicians are important additional sources of information but none fully capture what is meant by the *patients'* QOL. We would like to suggest that, whenever one has to decide about patients' QOL, the patients themselves should be asked, and in a way that allows for their self-determination. We, as researchers, physicians and mental health professionals, should listen carefully to what the patients have to say and not decide in advance by giving them only the option of pre-structured measurements. Furthermore, we wish to emphasize the importance of the cross-cultural aspect, which our new measure is suitable for investigating.

Acknowledgments

We wish to thank Dr. A. Loidl and Sandoz Pharma Ltd. in Basel, Switzerland, for their commitment and generosity, which enabled us to carry out this study. We also wish to thank the interviewers, nurses, physicians, statisticians and administrators for their fruitful cooperation.

References

Bar-on D, Amir M (1983) Re-examining quality of life of hypertensives: a new, self-structured measure. Am J Hypertension 6:S62–S66

Croog SH, Levine S, Testa MA, Brown B, Bulpitt CJ, Jenkins CD, Klerman GL, Williams GH (1986) The effect on antihypertensive therapy on the quality of life. New Engl Med 314:1657–1664

Frankenhauser M, Gardell B (1976) Underload and overload in working life: Outline of a multidisciplinary approach. J Human Stress 2:35–46

Golembiewski RT, Billingsley K, Yeager S (1976) Measuring change and persistence in human affairs: Types of change generated by OD designs. J Appl Behav Sci 12:133–157

Holmes T, Raye R (1967) The Social Readjustment Rating Scale. J Psychosomatic Res 11:213–218

Kobassa SC (1979) Stressful life events, personality and health: An inquiry into health. J Personality Social Psychol 37:1–11

Lubin B, Himmelstein P (1976) Reliability of the depression adjective check list. Perceptual Motor Skills 43:1037–1038

Rhodewalt F, Augustdottir S (1986) On the relationship of hardiness of the Type A behavior: Perception of life events versus coping with life events. J Res Personality 18:212–223

Siegriest J, Matschinger H, Motz W (1987) Untreated hypertensives and their quality of life. J Hypertension 5:S15–S20

Smoller-Wasserheil S, Blaufox DM, Oberman A, Davis BR, Swencionis C, O'Connell Knerr M, Hawkins CM, Landford HG (1991) Effect of antihypertensives on sexual function and quality of life: The TAIM study. Ann Internal Med 114:613–620

Testa MA, Anderson RB, Nackley JF, Hollenberg NK (1993) Quality of Life and Antihypertensive Therapy in Men. New Engl J Med 328:907–913

Testa MA, Hollenberg NK, Anderson RB, Williams GH (1991) Assessment of Quality of Life by patients and spouses during antihypertensive therapy with atenolol and nifedipine gastrointestinal therapeutic system. Am J Hypertension 4:363–373

Weingartner H, Grafman J, Boutelle W, Kaye W, Martin PR (1983) Forms of memory failure. Science 221:380–382

Yodfat Y, Cristal N (1993) A multicenter, double-blind, randomized, placebo-controlled study of Isradipine and Methyldopa as monotherapy or in combination with Captopril in the treatment of hypertension. Am J Hypertension 6:S57–S61

Subjective Quality of Life Assessment in Therapeutic Trials: Presentation of a New Instrument in France (SQLP: Subjective Quality of Life Profile) and First Results

A. Dazord, P. Gerin and *J.P. Boissel*

Summary

In therapeutic trials, quality of life studies are usually based on a health model which results in a restrictive view. Therefore, it is important to clearly define the concept of the quality of life, since ambiguous concepts can alter the results. The key to this problem is the clear distinction between the two components of the quality of life, i.e., subjective and objective. The latter component is the only one considered in the current medical approach.

The use of the subjective quality of life introduces a number of methodological problems not found when the objective quality of life is assessed, and thus requires a specific model which can be derived from the model of "life goals" used by sociologists. This model is presented here and illustrated with some results obtained with a new questionnaire, the Subjective Quality of Life Profile (SQLP). We suggest that both subjective and objective quality of life studies should be considered in order to emphasize the humanistic approach to therapeutic indications.

Introduction

The concept of the quality of life is complex, and many misunderstandings and difficulties encountered with quality of life studies in therapeutic trials arise when it is uncertain which aspect of the concept is being considered, i.e., the *objective* aspect of everyday life (ranging from health status to material considerations, including functional capabilities), or the *subjective* aspect (from the subject's own inner experience), or both. We should, therefore, speak of either the *objective quality of life* or the *subjective quality of life,* and use the general term *quality of life* only when both aspects are being considered.

The study of the objective quality of life is possible with existing methods or instruments, but the study of the subjective quality of life introduces new problems for which inadequate solutions exist. For this reason the following presentation focuses on the study of the subjective quality of life only, which does not, in any way, imply that the objective quality of life is unimportant.

Most of the instruments that have been developed focus on the assessment of health, as their names suggest: e.g., Sickness Impact Profile (SIP), Notting-

J. Orley, W. Kuyken (Eds.)
Quality of Life Assessment:
International Perspectives

ham Health Profile (NHP), McMaster Health Index Questionnaire (MHIQ; Bergner 1987; McEwen 1987; Chambers 1987). The NHP incorporates a subjective measure of health indicators, and the MHIQ includes an evaluation of the degree of satisfaction related to the various indicators. The Anamnestic Comparative Self-Assessment (ASCA) scale introduces a purely subjective approach to the assessment (Bernheim and Buyse 1983), and although the Purposes in Life (PIL) questionnaire introduces the concept of the "purpose in life," it has not been used in the field of therapeutic trials (Crumbaugh 1968). The Ferrans and Powers (Cella and Tulsky 1991) Quality of Life Index (FPQLI) and our Subjective Quality of Life Questionnaire (Gerin et al. 1992) are among the few questionnaires that systematically rate the degrees of both satisfaction and importance for all the items considered.

The second important point to consider is the fact that the concept of the quality of life is fundamentally diverse. Psychologists accept that the subjective quality of life is multi-dimensional, and, moreover, this is apparent in the assessments made by sociologists (Andrews and Witney 1976). Satisfaction and dissatisfaction experienced in different domains of life cannot be added together, algebraically, as they are not situated on the same continuum; therefore, the subjective quality of life can be considered to be multifactorial (Gerin et al. 1989, 1990). The presentation of results is therefore more appropriate in the form of *profiles* rather than *indices.* Although a profile is a somewhat simplistic representation of the real situation, it gives a more reliable image of the reality than an index, as it reflects the complexity of the concept.

In the field of health, quality of life studies may have one of two main aim. The first is to evaluate the effects of treatment(s) on the patients' quality of life. This implies studying whether or not changes in quality of life are different in patients receiving treatments than in control groups. The second aim is to describe and assess the patients' state in abnormal situations (e.g., clinical pathology or psychosocial disorder), to get a better knowledge of their needs. Clinical experience shows that it is the combination of clinical changes with the personal values of the subject which causes the changes in the subjective quality of life. The secondary effects of a treatment will not be experienced in the same way by different patients, depending on their personality. Thus, it is important to explain the changes in the subjective quality of life if we wish to optimize the choice of treatments.

Methods

The Questionnaire

The questionnaire that we developed (Subjective Quality of Life Profile; SLQP; Fig. 1) is derived from a model which uses the concept of "goals" in a very broad sense, so as to encompass wishes, expectations and drives, and which emphasizes that the most meaningful parameter is not the distance itself, but the way this distance is experienced by the individual, i.e., the subjective weight. This subjective weight depends on several factors, such as: 1) the *importance* attributed to each goal by the subject; 2) the individual's *tolerance* of the distance between his/her position and his/her goals, 3) his/her *ability to cope* with this distance, and in particular, to alter the importance attributed, i.e., change his/her values.

The first aim of this questionnaire was to make possible a comprehensive exploration of *the main domains of life*. These domains are:

1) *Functional life*. This area is well known to physicians since, when it is altered, the corresponding variables are transformed into symptoms of physical and mental illness. The first domain thus concerns both physical and mental *health*. All types of functions are considered: motor, psychological, sensory, sexual, sleep, digestion, pain, etc. This is the main domain taken into consideration by the majority of instruments currently available.

2) *Social life*. Social life can be subdivided into relationships (with other, friends, relatives, etc.), social roles, and interest in the exterior world.

3) *Material life*. Material life covers variables such as income, housing, etc.

4) *Spiritual life*. This domain of life is seldom explored with current instruments, although its importance for a number of subjects in certain cultures has been demonstrated. The importance may vary with the evolution of severe diseases and it is, therefore, a significant, but difficult domain of life to assess. Spiritual life is taken in its broadest sense, not only in the sense of the "ability to live esthetic or religious experiences," but also in the sense of meditation, thinking, reading, etc., and is even extended to so-called "future orientation," i.e., expectations, purposes in life, etc. (Joyce 1987).

5) *Unforeseen domains*. Studies which are to be carried out in different sociocultural backgrounds in various countries must be designed to be able to assess unforeseen domains, or at least some variables, which may be important to other cultures or to certain individuals and which cannot all be included in a questionnaire. Even if researchers were able to identify them all, their inclusion would result in a prohibitively long questionnaire, and the use of items which are important from our own point of view may lead to a tautological situation.

Naturally, it is important not to miss these unforeseen, important data. We have, therefore, included a set of open-ended questions to solve this dilemma. An example of this type of question is; "What is the most important (or the most satisfying, or the most worrying) thing in your current life?"

6) *Global assessments*. Several domains are investigated to determine the overall subjective quality of life, e.g., humour, subjective evaluation of the treatment, and relationships with health care personnel. The importance of the therapeutic alliance is not just restricted to the psychotherapeutic field (Luborsky et al. 1983).

The choice of the measures to be used for the various items is a problem. Most of the current instruments do not consider this problem because they

The items included in the questionnaire are:

1. With regard to your physical ability to perform everyday movements, (i.e., lifting things, bending over, washing and dressing yourself, climbing stairs, etc.):
2. With regard to your ability to get out and about outside the home:
3. With regard to your overall fitness, during the day:
4. With regard to feeling (or not feeling) aches and/or pains in some parts of your body:
5. With regard to the way you digest your food:
6. With regard to sleep:
7. With regard to your sexuality:
8. With regard to your ability to think and concentrate:
9. With regard to your eyesight:
10. With regard to your hearing:
11. With regard to your income:
12. With regard to your being able to carry out daily activities, either domestic (housework, maintenance) or professional (outside the home):
13. With regard to the fact that you have (or do not have) a professional activity:
14. With regard to any possible concern that you may have about your health:
15. With regard to what is going on in the world (economically, socially, politically):
16. With regard to what you can (or cannot) eat:
17. With regard to what you can (or cannot) drink:
18. With regard to your weight:
19. With regard to your relationships with other people in general:
20. With regard to your religious beliefs/faith:
21. With regard to your participation (or not) in various activities (cultural, religious, unions):
22. With regard to the time you spend (or do not spend) with friends:
23. With regard to the relationships that you have (or do not have) with your family
24. With regard to a special relationship with somebody
25. In terms of your activities, both at home and at work:
26. With regard to any hobbies or activities that you might have (for example: sport, do-it-yourself, painting):
27. With regard to other peoples' attitudes towards you:
28. With regard to your physical appearance (e.g. when you see yourself in a mirror):
29. With regard to the material conditions of your daily life:
30. With regard to your inner life (reflections, reading, meditation, etc.):
31. With regard to the relationships that you have (or do not have) with your father and mother:
32. With regard to the relationships that you have (or do not have) with your children:
33. With regard to the fact that you feel free (or absolutely not):

Fig. 1. Subjective Quality of Life Profile (SQLP Questionnaire)

focus on the assessment of the objective quality on life only. In our proposed model of the subjective quality of life, a set of specific measures, rather than a single type of measure, are performed.

1) *Ability (or change).* A subject's own assessment of his/her ability or inability with respect to any item provides information concerning his/her "objective" state.

2) *Degree of satisfaction.* The degree of satisfaction corresponding to each domain of life is a direct and simple measure for evaluating what the subject is

Questions Asked for Each Item

*Are you:
- O Very dissatisfied
- O Slightly dissatisfied
- O Indifferent
- O Mildly satisfied
- O Very satisfied

*How important is this to you
- O Unimportant
- O Fairly important
- O Very important

*In the coming months do you expect that this will:
- O Change in a very unfavourable direction
- O Change in a fairly unfavourable direction
- O Not change
- O Change in a fairly favourable direction
- O Change in a very favourable direction

*Have you been able to cope with the difficulty you have encountered with regard to...
- O Not at all
- O Not well enough
- O Reasonably well
- O Very well

Is there something else which seems to be important to you that has not been mentioned here?:....

Fig. 1 (continued)

experiencing. This measure is essential for the subjective quality of life assessment, although the current instruments rarely use it and then only for a few items.

3) *Importance attributed.* A direct assessment of the subjective importance attributed to the various domains of life by the individual is possible, but the majority of existing instruments do not do this. The personal values of the individual, and any changes relating to them during treatment or disease, are identified by this assessment. This type of measure is thus useful if we want to explain the level of the subjective quality of life and/or its changes.

4) *Change anticipated.* The direct assessment, at the beginning of treatment, of the degree of change *anticipated* for each domain allows a comparison with the degree of change actually *experienced* by the subjects (after the treatment).

5) *Ability to cope.* A subject's ability to cope with difficulties encountered is another important factor in the relationship between the objective and subjective quality of life. The assessment of this is, therefore, important when changes in the subjective quality of life are to be explained, but such an assessment is not necessary for each domain.

6) *Global measures.* A global assessment of the subjective quality of life through direct questions (e.g., "How happy are you?"), although lacking in sensitivity, may be useful in certain situations. *A global subjective assessment of the treatment* and the degree of confidence in the health care personnel can also be added.

Subjects

This questionnaire was validated on several sample populations: Sample 1) 700 hypertensive patients randomly allocated to receive as monotherapy either a combination of two diuretics, a beta blocker, a calcium antagonist, or an angiotension-converting enzyme inhibitor; Sample 2) 800 diabetic patients randomly allocated to receive either a classical form of insulin or a pen-injection; Sample 3) 40 patients who had recently suffered from an acute myocardial infarction and who had been enrolled in a study to receive prolonged treatment with heparin; Sample 4) 65 depressed patients (depression being assessed by MADRS; Montgomery and Asberg 1979) recently hospitalized in a psychiatric department, or in a general hospital curing alcoholic patients; and Sample 5) 50 patients with severe lung cancer.

Statistical Analyses

When descriptive studies are performed, we used the chi square test for comparisons of proportions. The scoring system requires the use of a non-parametric test (e.g., Wilcoxon signed rank test) to estimate, for instance (Sample 3), the significance of the difference between responses and the anticipated and the observed changes (Siegel 1956) or a Spearman rho to estimate correlations. The usual level of significance ($p = 0.05$) is generally not used, due to the number of repeated tests and, from Bonferroni's inequality, we usually calculate that we should use $p = < 0.01$. Information concerning the patient's quality of life structure is derived from factorial analysis (principal component analysis or multiple correspondence analysis; Benzecri 1979).

When clinical trials are performed (Samples 1 and 2) the subjective quality of life data are compared between the groups, using a conventional ANOVA approach and a specific statistical analytical approach developed for the SQLP questionnaire. Scheffe's constants are computed to compare the groups in a pairwise manner (Scheffe 1959). The alpha level is set at 0.05 (two-tailed). The theoretical number of subjects required to detect a significant difference (with alpha = 0.05 and beta = 0.10) is calculated for all items, using multivariate analyses (ANCOVA) and considering several factors, i.e., "importance attributed" to the item, sex, age class as covariables and random allocation into the different subgroups (Gerin et al. 1992).

Validation Studies

The validation of the questionnaire has been described in detail elsewhere (Gerin et al. 1991). Internal consistency was estimated by split-half correlation (0.93) and Cronbach alpha (0.90). Reliability was estimated by test-retest (Spearman rho was used to evaluate the correlation between the questions concerning "the importance attributed to" at the first evaluation and one month later; it ranged around 0.5 with $p < 0.0005$).

In the depressed patients (Sample 4) we are able to detect a meaningful correlation between the MADRS score (which is a depression scale filled out by the clinician) and both the global score of satisfaction at the SQLP and the sum of all satisfactions (rho = 0.40, $p < 0.001$). In another study with lung cancer patients we found a clear correlation (rho = 0.61, $p = 0.05$) between the Karnofsky index, which is a physician evaluation of the patient's autonomy (Karnofsky et al. 1949), and the patients' reported satisfaction related to their daily activities.

The acceptability of the questionnaire is also quite satisfactory since, in most studies, more than 90% of the subjects returned the questionnaire.

Results

Quality of Life and Medical Treatments

Quality of life has become a relevant measure of efficacy in clinical studies. It may help to differentiate between different therapies or describe outcomes in different treatment modalities.

Antihypertensive Treatments

A study performed on 700 asymptomatic patients (Sample 1, above) compared the effects of four major classes of antihypertensive treatments. A global test for the differences in the quality of life scores at one month was highly significant ($p = 0.0001$), and this result was unchanged after adjustment for the items which initially showed an imbalance in favour of one group (i.e., general well-being, sleep, libido, daily life). The global satisfaction was greater in this group after adjustment for importance attributed to and discomfort felt at base line, with p-values ranging from 0.033 to 0.0005. After further adjustment for the base line imbalances mentioned above, the differences for six of these items remained statistically significant. At nine months, however, these differences disappeared and the global test was no longer significant ($p = 0.13$).

Insulin Treatments

We compared the effects of regular insulin and pen-injection (Sample 2) in 800 patients. After adjustment for the items which initially showed an imbalance in favour of the pen-injection group, this study showed a statistical difference concerning the degree of satisfaction in favour of the pen-injection for three items: going out or moving around ($p<0.0001$), daily activities ($p = 0.001$), and group activities ($p = 0.001$).

Heparin Treatment in Myocardial Infarction

In this study, the responses showed globally that there is an overall feeling of satisfaction on a 5-level scale ranging from -2 (very dissatisfatied) to $+2$ (very satisfied). The items for which the greatest satisfaction was expressed were not related to patients' symptoms but to their relationships (e.g., with family and friends, 0.6) and digestion, sleep, and concentration (0.8, 0.6, and 1).

It is usually assumed that the satisfaction or dissatisfaction felt for a given item can be explained by the direction of change, i.e., positive or negative, and therefore a strong correlation should be observed. However, in this study this was not the case for all items (Table 1), since strong negative correlations were observed between the change and the degree of satisfaction or dissatisfaction felt for the major symptoms of pain, fatigue, and the consequences of these (i.e., concern about health). The differences between the anticipated changes (on a 5-level scale ranging from -2 to $+2$) and those actually experienced (on the same scale) were calculated as the difference in these scores for each item. Using the Wilcoxon signed rank test we found that the strongest and statistically significant ($p = 0.00003$) deception concerned anginal pain, with a value of -1.6, although the patients had noted a clear improvement. Fatigue and concern about health also had negative values which were close to the level of significance ($p = 0.015$). Therefore, the most important result from this study concerns the way in which the patients experienced the changes in their major symptoms, i.e., anginal pain and fatigue. Disappointment – due to the fact

Table 1. Paradoxical dissatisfaction

Item	Difference between expected and actual changes	Correlation between changes and (dis)satisfaction Spearman rho
Pain	−1.6**	−0.4
Fatigue	−0.2*	−0.6
Concern about health	−0.55*	−0.7
Mobility	0.53	0.75
Digestion	0.13	0.6
Others' attitudes	0.43	0.7
Sleep	0.1	0.7
Libido	0.67	0.8
Relationships in general	0.27	0.65
Relationships with friends	0	0.55
Relationships with family	0.06	0.4

* $p = 0.01$; ** $p<0.0001$

that the effective change that was experienced did not match up to the anticipated change – can explain what may seem to be a paradoxical impairment of the subjective quality of life (i.e., a negative degree of satisfaction) concomitant with an improvement in the objective quality of life (i.e., a positive change in the degreee of ability).

Special Populations and Approaches to Quality of Life

Physicians are expected to use their empathic knowledge of their patient's personality (the patient's values) in the decision-making process concerning choice of treatment, so as to favour the patient's subjective quality of life. This approach can be developed further, with the aim of describing the interactions between a treatment and the patient's personality. Joyce (1987) suggested that it would be useful to be able to identify those subjects who have a higher probability of benefiting from favourable, subjective results which are known not to be applicable to everybody. For example, in the aforementioned comparative trial of two different types of treatments for diabetic patients, it was found that the treatment which was easier to use away from home (insulin pen-injection) was preferred by those subjects who were involved in external activities. On the other hand, patients suffering from lung cancer (Sample 5), although saying their pain was quite important, described their leisure time as the domain where they were the most dissatisfied, and not their physical health.

Thus, it can be necessary to define the typology of patients in terms of their values, i.e., the importance they attribute to each domain of their life, so that the effects of a given treatment on the subjective quality of life can be studied for each type of patient. These types of studies can be performed using multifactorial analysis.

Sample 4 (see Methods section) was composed of 65 depressed patients, 70% of whom were alcoholic. The profiles obtained were significantly different from those found in all three other samples populations. Concerning the degree of satisfaction or dissatisfaction, for instance, these patients were indifferent to most domains. However, a very clear dissatisfaction was related to health problems, fatigue, and pain. The second striking finding concerned the degree of change anticipated: it did not allow discrimination between the various domains, and it was significantly much higher (mean = 1.45 compared to 0.4 for patients with myocardial infarction, $p < 0.0001$, on a 5-level scale ranging from -2 to $+2$). Multiple correspondence analysis showed that alcoholic depressed patients clearly differed from non-alcoholic depressed patients; active variables were constituted by variables related to importance attributed. Two axes emerged: the first (20% of total inertia) was related to material life and distinguished the alcoholic patients who attributed great importance to it, whereas non-alcoholic depressed subjects did not. The second axis represented 7% of total inertia and distinguished between those who attributed great importance to relationships in general, and group activities (the alcoholic patients), versus those who did not (the non-alcoholic depressed patients).

Conclusion

Thus, our SQLP questionnaire, which takes into account the abilities of or changes experienced by the patients, as well as their degree of satisfaction, the importance they attributed to the various domains of life, and their expectations concerning these various domains, offers several interesting findings:

1) it provides different profiles for different populations;
2) it allows detection, after treatments, of some very specific, sometimes unexpected, changes;
3) it provides a possible explanation of some of these quality of life changes by, for instance the initial typology (personality) of the patients or by the degree of their expectations.

Therefore, we expect that this tool will help physicians in their decision-making process concerning choice of treatments.

References

Andrews FM, Witney SB (1976) Social indicators of well-being: American's perception of life quality. New York, Plenum Press

Benzecri JP (1979) L'analyse des données. Dunod 3° ed

Bergner M (1987) Development, testing and use of the Sickness Impact Profile. In: Walker SR, Rosser RM (eds) Quality of life: assessment and application. MTP Press Limited, Lancaster, Boston, The Hague, Dordrecht

Bernheim JL, Buyse M (1983) The anamnestic comparative self-assessment for measuring the subjective quality of life of cancer patients. J Psychol Soc 14:25.38

Cella DF, Tulsky DS (1991) Measuring quality of life today: methodological aspects (Appendix pp 209–232). Oncology 4:29–38

Chambers LW (1987) The McMaster Health Index questionnaire: an update. In: Walker SR, Rosser RM (eds) Quality of life: assessment and application. MTP Press Limited, Lancaster, Boston, The Hague, Dordrecht

Crumbaugh JC (1968) Cross-validation of Purpose-in-life Test based on Frankl's concepts. J Individ Psychol 24:74–81

Gerin P, Dazord A, Boissel JP, Hanauer MT, Moleur P, Chauvin F (1989) L'evaluation de la qualité de la vie dans les essais thérapeutiques. Aspects conceptuels et présentation d'un questionnaire. Thérapie 44:355–364

Gerin P, Dazord A, Boissel JP, Hanauer MT (1990) Assessment of quality of life in therapeutic trials. In: Strauch G, Husson JM (eds) Recent trends in clinical pharmacology. EDITIONS INSERM, 186:143–163

Gerin P, Dazord A, Cialdella P, Leizorovicz A, Boissel JP, and the OCAPI Research Group (1991) Le questionnaire< <Profil de la Qualité de la Vie Subjective> >(PQVS). Premiers éléments de validation. Thérapie 46:131–138

Gerin P, Dazord A, Boissel JP, Chifflet R (1992) Quality of life assessment in therapeutic trials: rationale for and presentation of a more appropriate instrument. Fund Clin Pharmacol 6:263–276

Joyce CRB (1987) Quality of life: the state of the art in clinical assessment. In: Walker SR, Rosser RM (eds) Quality of life: assessment and application. MTP Press, Limited, Lancaster, Boston, The Hague, Dordrecht

Karnofsky DA, Burchenal JH (1949) The clinical evaluation of chemotherapeutic agents against cancer. In: McLeod CM (ed) Evaluation of chemotherapeutic agents. New York, Columbia University Press

Luborsky L, Crits-Cristoph P, Alexander L, Margolis M, Cohen M (1983) Two helping alliance methods of predicting outcomes of psychotherapy: a counting signs versus a global rating method. J Nervous Mental Dis 171:590–603

McEwen J (1987) The Nottingham Health Profile: In: Walker SR, Rosser RM (eds) Quality of life: assessment and application. MTP Press Limited, Lancaster, Boston, The Hague, Dordrecht

Montgomery SA, Asberg M (1979) A new depression scale designed to be sensitive to change. Brit J Psychiat 134:382–389

Scheffé H (1959) The analysis of variance. New York, Wiley

Siegel S (1956) Nonparametric statistics for behavioral sciences. MCGraw-Hill, New York

Subject Index

MIX
Papier aus verantwortungsvollen Quellen
Paper from responsible sources
FSC® C105338

If you have any concerns about our products,
you can contact us on
ProductSafety@springernature.com

In case Publisher is established outside the EU,
the EU authorized representative is:
Springer Nature Customer Service Center GmbH
Europaplatz 3, 69115 Heidelberg, Germany

Printed by Libri Plureos GmbH
in Hamburg, Germany